Beginner's Guide to Essential Oils and Herbal Tinctures: DIY Natural Remedies with Herbs, Aromatherapy Recipes, Infused Oils, and Much More!

Homesteading Freedom

Kathy Wyatt

Published by CiJiRO Publishing, 2020.

While every precaution has been taken in the preparation of this book, the publisher assumes no responsibility for errors or omissions, or for damages resulting from the use of the information contained herein.

BEGINNER'S GUIDE TO ESSENTIAL OILS AND HERBAL TINCTURES: DIY NATURAL REMEDIES WITH HERBS, AROMATHERAPY RECIPES, INFUSED OILS, AND MUCH MORE!

First edition. March 31, 2020.

Copyright © 2020 Kathy Wyatt.

ISBN: 978-1386601227

Written by Kathy Wyatt.

Beginner's Guide to Essential Oils and Herbal Tinctures

DIY Natural Remedies with Herbs, Aromatherapy Recipes, Infused Oils, and Much More!

Kathy Wyatt

© 2017

The trademarks that are used are without any consent, and the publication of the trademark is without permission or backing by the trademark owner. All trademarks and brands within this book are for clarifying purposes only and are the owned by the owners themselves, not affiliated with this document.

Introduction

In this book you'll learn everything you need to know for essential oils and herbal tinctures to help you with a variety of ailments. There are many uses for both essential oils and herbal tinctures, and using these amazing remedies and blends shouldn't be hard. This book strives to make it easy to use essential oils, tinctures, and more to help you with the various problems in your life. You'll learn about salves, infused oil for cooking, balms and even beauty products that can be made as well. There are many ways to use herbs to help better your health, mentally, emotionally and physically. There's no reason to rely on chemical based products or medication.

;

Chapter 1: What an Essential Oil Is

You may be wondering what essential oils actually are, and that's exactly what will be covered in this chapter. Before you start using essential oils, you need to know about them if you wish to use them safely and get the desired results. In short, essential oils are a highly concentrated oil that is taken from a plant, and they do this by using a still. If you want to buy your own still to make your own essential oils, there will be a still buying guide later on in this book so stay tuned! Still, many people feel that buying their essential oils is best because it is cheaper in the short run and much easier.

Distillation

Distillation in either water or steam is how you get essential oils, but the part of the plant that you use for this will depend on the essential oil you are trying to make. In different essential oils you will use different parts, but they can be made from the roots, leaves, flowers and stems. You can even make some essential oils from bark. Once the distillation is finished, you'll have a highly concentrated oil that will have the scent and characteristics. It will certainly keep the healing properties that the plant had.

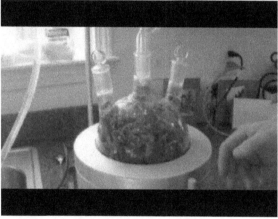

Figure 1: essential oil distiller

Therapeutic Properties

Aromatherapy is the most common application for essential oils, but they are known to be therapeutic overall. Many essential oils are also antiseptic, meaning that they will reduce the risk of infection once applied topically. They also are believed to have an uplifting effect on a person's mind. There is no official grading system, but if the essential oil is pure then it should have all of its therapeutic qualities. When you're looking for a "100% pure essential oil" then that means you're looking for a single essential oil and not a blend of essential oils or carrier oils. However, you'll have some companies that have fillers, chemical aromas and additives, so just make sure that you are getting your essential oils from a respectable company.

Are they Fragrances?

No, essential oils aren't the same as fragrance oils or perfumes. Perfume oils are created artificially. Essential oils are an all-natural product. Fragrances do not have the same therapeutic benefits that natural essential oils have. You cannot use fragrances for aromatherapy for this reason. You'll mostly use fragrances for soap making, candle making, cosmetics and perfumes.

Pure Oil vs an Oil Blend

You can buy essential oils in a pure form, which again is a single essential oil or you can get a blend. A blend has several essential oils and often a carrier oil. Essential oil blends can be made or bought. A blend is designed to achieve a certain purpose, and this book will teach you how to make your own blends. When you make your own blends you have control over every ingredient that goes into it to make sure that you're getting exactly what you want.

Essential Oil Storage & Safety

You should store essential oils in a closed bottle, and it should be in a cool place out of direct sunlight. Make sure that it isn't in the reach of pets or children. You should never put essential oils in your nose, ears or inside your eyes. Before using essential oils, make sure to dilute them properly.

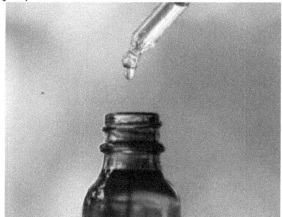

Chapter 2: Essential Oil Myths

Before we get into how essential oils are made and how to use them, you should know a few of the common myths about essential oils. If you don't know what is and isn't true, then you won't be able to use essential oils properly. Let's cover some of the most basic myths and what the truth actually is.

Better Brands

It's a myth that there are better brands of essential oils. Trying to figure out the best oil is completely subjective. It can be a pure oil and still be a flat one, which is just like flat wine. However, some people will prefer quantity over artistry as well, which makes it even more difficult to figure out what brand would be "best". If you are looking for an essential fragrance, you'll be looking for affordability. You won't be looking for layered fragrance.

Labels Are Important

As you'll learn more in the next chapter, "therapeutic grade" isn't important for a label because there is no general labeling system. These labels are just marketing ploys, so you won't want to fall into them.

There are No "Absolutes"

Essential oils are something that is distilled or in the case of citrus it's pressed. However, there are floral oils that are considered to be essential oils. These are not able to be distilled because they are too delicate. Instead, they are separated with a solvent, making them an absolute. They will be called an essential oil and can be used in the same way, but they are not exactly the same.

Essential Oils are Destroyed by Heat

Essential oils are not destroyed by heat like many people will try to tell you. Think about it this way. Essential oils are made with a heat based diffuser, so of course they can handle heat. It's still best to choose a cool, dark storage space to help to prolong the lifespan. Light will degrade the essential oil over time. Violet glass will block visible light rays, so it's a great way to store essential oils too.

Nutrition Facts are Important

Many people seem to think that if an essential oil is top quality then it'll have a nutrition facts section on the label. This isn't true, and it's a false line of logic. They are just trying to tell you it's pure to eat so it is the best type of essential oil. This is just another marketing ploy.

Standardization is Still Pure

This is where an essential oil is mixed with another compound, and people like to think that this isn't the same as adulteration of an essential oil. Since that would be mixing it with a different compound, this is virtually the same thing. It still leaves you without a pure essential oil, but that doesn't mean they won't work. It just means that they won't work as well, and they're certainly not safe to ingest. Of course, it's also debatable that essential oils are safe to ingest in the first place.

Chapter 3: Essential Oil Extraction

Everyone wants to know how to make essential oils at home, but without a still it's almost impossible. However, to understand why you need to understand the extraction process. Essential oils are powerful because they are concentrated forms of oil found in a plant, so even if you could extract the oil yourself it would take a lot of plant material to produce an extremely small amount of oil which makes it quite difficult to secure the amount of plant material that would be needed.

Why Method is Important

If you want to buy quality oils, you need to know a little about the extraction method as well. In short, the extraction method will tell you how good the essential oil is. The way in which an essential oil is distilled can affect how volatile it is, the aroma and even the strength. Here are a few examples.

- **Distilled Patchouli:** This is prized for the aroma that it has which is richer than a type that is non-distilled.
- **Distilled Citrus:** This will be less stable than an expressed oil even if it's the same oil. However, that isn't always a bad thing. It's just something that you need to keep in mind. For example, distilled citrus is best for topical application because it reduces photo-toxicity
- **C02 Extracts:** These include myrrh and frankincense will have more beneficial molecules than one that are distilled.

You won't always have an option on which type of essential oil that you're going to buy, but there are times that you'll want to research it and try to make an educated decision on which will work best for your needs. However, most essential oils are fine for almost all remedies. You won't find that the blends in this book require a preference.

Extraction Methods

Different manufacturers will use different types of extraction methods. In this section you'll find the most three common extraction methods for essential oils.

- **Distillation:** This will employ either steam or water to separate the oil from the plant matter. This takes place in a large still, and the still has a connecting pipe that goes to a condenser. The finished essential oil is then siphoned. A long, slow heating process is used for the best essential oils.
- **CO2 Extraction:** This uses carbon dioxide or supercritical carbon dioxide to separate the plant matter for the essential oil. There isn't any heating involved so the oil is unaltered and pure. The product is close to its original plant oil as it can get, and it produces a very pure form of an essential oil.
- **Expression:** This is often called cold pressing, and it's usually used for citrus essential oils. The oil is concentrated inside the fruit skin, so pressing after heating the rinds to about 120 degrees F ensures that the fragrance is maintained.

Buying Your Own Still

Though it is cheaper in the short run and by far easier, some people still may be interested in buying their own still to make essential oils. Remember that you should make sure you are getting a quality still, and you'll want to get it from a respectable online supplier. Some people choose to make their own, but it can be dangerous if made improperly so this is not recommended. A simple steam still will cost you anywhere from $200-$500. This is the best type of still to use when trying to make your own essential oils at home.

Chapter 4: Single Essential Oils

There are countless essential oils that you can buy, and which ones you buy will depend on what applications you plan to use them for. However, there are some basic essential oils to start with that are often used on their own. That's what this chapter is dedicated to so that you know what essential oils to experiment with before learning to make your own blends.

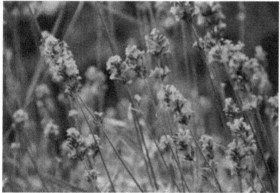

Lavender Essential Oil

When most people think of essential oils, one of the first essential oils they think of is lavender. It's a common scent that's used in so many things that most people grow up with it even if they're nowhere near lavender fields. This is one of the most popular essential oils, and not only because of its scent. Lavender is a versatile essential oil that promotes calming and relaxation.

You can use it for body mists, shampoos, and conditioners, hair mists, in diffusers or topically with a carrier oil. You can apply it topically to help with insect bites, skin rashes, acne, and minor burns when used for a carrier oil. If you put a few drops in a bath, then it can help to sooth your nerves. It can also help to alleviate respiratory infections and sinus issues when used in a diffuser. When you use lavender oil on sachets it can help to keep moths away as well.

Tea Tree Essential Oil

This is considered a medicine cabinet essential, so it's definitely an essential oil to start with. It can be used topically with a carrier oil to treat athlete's foot, nail fungus, warts, insect bites, cold sores, acne, and even eczema. When you add a few drops to an unscented shampoo then it can help with psoriasis as well as dandruff. It can also treat head lice when used in shampoo as well. You can create a disinfectant spray by adding a few drops of tea tree essential oil to water and placing it in a misting bottle as well. A few drops around the pet bed will help to keep fleas at bay as well.

Lemon Essential Oil

This is yet another versatile essential oil that is a home staple. You can make an antibacterial scour with coarse salt, baking soda and a few drops of lemon essential oil. This works great for butcher blocks as well as cutting boards. When you add a few drops to a glass of water, you can gargle with it to relieve bad breath as well. Reduce dandruff by adding some to unscented shampoo. It can even help to get rid of your anxiety and stress if you add a few drops to a diffuser or even to a bath. It makes a great antimicrobial hand sanitizer when you add it to aloe gel as well. Just make sure to blend well! You should avoid the sun for twelve to twenty-four hours after applying this essential oil topically.

Peppermint Essential Oil

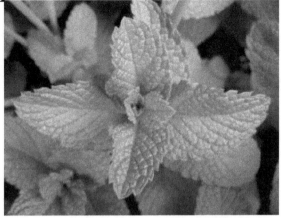

If you're having an upset stomach or experiencing nausea, then you can add a few drops of peppermint essential oil to a carrier oil of your choice to hand massage it onto your stomach. If you have a pet with a tick under their skin, add undiluted peppermint essential oil to the spot which will draw it out so that you can kill it. if you need to find a way to help your overheated, tired feet then add a few drops to cool water and soak your feet. Adding it to a spray bottle full of water will help with odors. If you add it to cracks in the walls, then it can help to deter spiders and rodents as well.

Eucalyptus Essential Oil

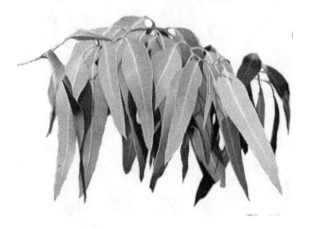

If you're having issues with chest congestion, then just diffuse some of this essential oil on its own or put it in a carrier oil and apply to the chest region. If you add a few drops to a compress it can help to ease the pain that comes from shingles. It will also help the healing process. It also had disinfectant properties by adding it to a spray bottle full of water you can use it around your home. It also works as an odor eliminator.

Clove Essential Oil

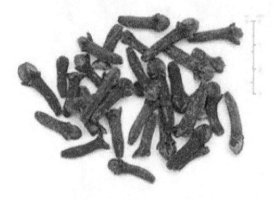

Clove is commonly used for dental issues. It can treat gum disease, cold sores, canker sores and even a toothache. Just make sure that it's diluted with a carrier oil that is able to be ingested. You should never apply it topically without it being diluted. It can be used for prickly heat rash, cuts and wounds, insect stings, insect bites, athlete's foot, and even bruises. You can also use it for ear aches by putting some on a cotton swab and tucking it right inside the ear canal. If you want to repel mosquitos just add a few drops in a diffuser. You can also get rid of fleas bay sprinkling a baking soda and clove essential oil mixture on carpets before vacuuming.

Chamomile Essential Oil

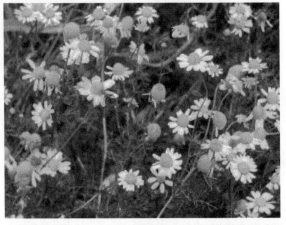

This is a soothing and gentle essential oil that can help with a variety of conditions other than just nerves and anxiety when added to a diffuser. When you apply it topically along with carrier oil it can help with wasp stings, bee stings, dermatitis, eczema, dry skin, boils, bruises and even cuts. When you put it in a diffuser it can help with depression, stress, anxiety and even insomnia.

Frankincense Essential Oil

You can use frankincense's essential oil or quite a while as well, and it has many topical application when used with a carrier oil. You can use it for scar tissue, cysts, insect bites, cuts, warts, boils and even acne. It can also help to alleviate stress as well as reduce migraines when used in a diffuser.

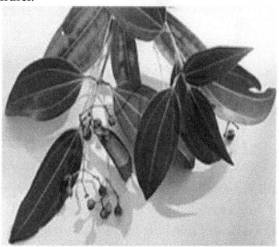

Grapefruit Essential Oil

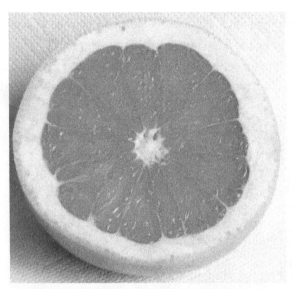

This is another multi-purpose essential oil that's great to start with. It has an uplifting and cheery scent, but when used with a carrier oil it can be used topically for a variety of things. It can be used for oily hair, oily skin, swollen lymph nodes, cellulite, tension headaches and migraine, and even acne. A few drops around a dog's bed will help to repel fleas as well. Just keep in mind that after applying topically you need to avoid the sun for twelve to twenty-four hours.

Oregano Essential Oil

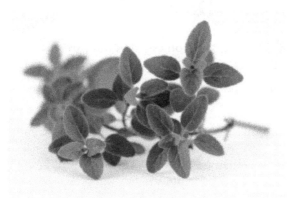

This essential oil is anti-parasitic, anti-microbial, anti-fungal and even anti-inflammatory. It also has antiseptic properties, and it can be used around your house as well as on your body. However, you should never use this undiluted. If you're nursing or pregnant avoid this essential oil as well. You can use it with a carrier oil to help with cysts, warts, shingles, sprains, athlete's foot, fungal infections, and bruises. When you dilute it in a spray bottle of water you use it as an anti-bacterial spray for around the house. It repels bugs, especially undiluted, by adding it to your bed. It'll repel fleas, mites, bed bugs, and lice.

Chapter 5: Further Essential Oil Break Down

You know a few of the most common essential oils now, but there are still more essential oils out there. In this chapter, you'll learn all about a few common ailments and the various essential oils that can help to address the issue.

For Age Spots

To understand why certain essential oils can help with age spots, you need to understand what causes them. When melanin is produced in excess, age spots can form. It can also be exposure to ultraviolet light, excess exposure to the sun, and the most likely spots are shoulders, hands, face, back and forearms.

- **Sandalwood Essential Oil:** This is great for age spots because it has skin regenerative properties while being an astringent and skin tonic naturally.
- **Frankincense Essential Oil:** You already know so many uses for frankincense, but you'll find that it can help with age spots as well.
- **Carrot Seed Essential Oil:** This is restorative for skin, and it helps with the regeneration of cells. It can help smooth over dry skin and lighten the skin as well as toning it.
- **Geranium Essential Oil:** This is great at normalizing sebum production which will diminish age spots. It will also tighten your skin and keep the elasticity in it. It can even help to improve blood circulation.
- **Myrrh Essential Oil:** This is great for age spots because it has anti-inflammatory properties while helping skin elasticity and firmness. It can help with rashes, sun damage, eczema, and chapped skin as well.
- **Patchouli Essential Oil:** This helps with new cell growth, and it can help with acne, eczema and psoriasis too.
- **Rose Essential Oil:** This is a powerful antimicrobial and anti-inflammatory. It helps to tone your skin, and it reduces stress which educe the stress hormone cortisol which wreaks havoc on your complexion.
- **Pomegranate Seed Oil:** This has a lot of antioxidants in it

that can help to reduce radical damage and even slow the aging process. It'll help with skin regeneration and increased elasticity.

- **Cypress Essential Oil:** This strengthens your skin while improving your blood circulation.

For Pain & Inflammation Relief

Pain and inflammation is best treated when the essential oil is used topically.

- **Sweet Marjoram Essential Oil:** This has a sedative effect that also works as an anti-inflammatory. It often helps with migraines, headaches, nerve pain, and even stomach cramps. It can help to relieve a toothache when the essential oil is placed around the sore tooth as well.
- **Eucalyptus Essential Oil:** This is a powerful essential oil for pain relief, and it can even help with blocked sinuses. It can help with muscle pain, joint pain, headaches and arthritis. It's an anti-inflammatory that also has antibacterial properties and antioxidants.
- **Peppermint Essential Oil:** This is an antispasmodic, which means it's great for intestinal problems as well as arthritis. It has anti-inflammatory and antimicrobial properties. It also contains a large amount of menthol which can help with muscular pains and aches as well as tension headaches.
- **Thyme Essential Oil:** This is great if you suffer from inflammation, muscle pains and backache. It has anti-inflammatory properties and it has an antispasmodic effect. It can help to reduce menstrual cramps too.
- **Clary Sage Essential Oil:** This helps with menstrual pain, muscle cramps, and it has muscle relaxing properties.
- **Juniper Essential Oil:** It relieves stiffness and it can numb pain in both joints and muscles. You can make a juniper berry compress with this essential oil as well, but it works great when made into an ointment.
- **Yarrow Essential Oil:** This helps with rheumatic pain as well as intestinal cramping when made into a tea. It can help to

reduce inflammation when applied topically as well.

- **Wintergreen Essential Oil:** This helps with chronic lower back pain, stiff joints and muscle aches.
- **Vetiver Essential Oil:** This is an anti-inflammatory and it has a soothing effect. It can help with muscular pain and headaches too.
- **Black Pepper Essential Oil:** This is great for pains and muscle aches, and it will help to increase blood circulation. It's also an anti-inflammatory and antibacterial. It's particularly helpful with shoulder aches and neck pain.
- **Rose Geranium Essential Oil:** This is great with muscle aches, knee pain and back aches. It's a good pain relief for nerve related conditions such as shingles as well.
- **Bergamot Essential Oil:** This is often used for headaches and anxiety, but it can help with some nerve pain as well.

For Acne

Sometimes it's difficult to make an essential oil blend for something as simple as acne, so try these single essential oils. Just mix them with a carrier oil and apply them topically. Just remember that a blend or cream usually will work better and quicker than a single essential oil.

- **Tea Tree Essential Oil:** This is great at fighting bacteria to get rid of blackheads and whiteheads. It's also great for a variety of skin infections.
- **Lemongrass Essential Oil:** This is great for your skin, and it'll help to reduce the appearance of acne quickly. It's a natural astringent, so you won't have oily skin when using this oil. It can also help to reduce acne scars too.
- **Basil Essential Oil:** This is great because it's an antimicrobial. It will reduce skin infections such as acne as well as inflammation.
- **Sandalwood Essential Oil:** This will boost the healthy appearance of your sin as an antiseptic, anti-inflammatory and astringent. It will lock in moisture as well as get rid of acne.
- **Chamomile Essential Oil:** If you're looking for the signs of acne to be reduced immediately, then this will help you to reduce the look of acne as well as treating it.

For Energy

Sometimes everyone needs a pick me up, but there are essential oils that can help to give you energy too. Try putting one of these in a diffuser instead of grabbing a cup of coffee next time.

- **Orange Essential Oil:** Citrus essential oils in general are a great way to give you a quick boost of energy and focus.
- **Cedarwood Essential Oil:** This is a calming essential oil but it will help to give you a better quality sleep which will make you feel energized come morning.
- **Spearmint Essential Oil:** This will help to boost your energy levels soon after you smell it, and peppermint can be used as well.
- **Cinnamon Essential Oil:** This has a warming infect and it improves energy levels when applied topically because it improves blood flow as well as blood sugar levels.
- **Lemon Essential Oil:** Once again a citrus essential oil boosts your mood and helps to boost your energy levels as well.

For Fleas

No one wants to deal with fleas, but it can be difficult to always use chemicals to get rid of them. These essential oils can get rid of fleas without having to expose you or your pets to harsh chemicals.

- **Citronella Essential Oil:** This essential oil is highly effective against most bugs, but it especially is effective against fleas and ticks.
- **Thyme Essential Oil:** Since this essential oil is a fungicide, bactericide and pesticide, it's a great way to get rid of fleas.
- **Cedarwood Essential Oil:** This is known as an insect repellent, and it's especially effective when you mix it with lemongrass and/or citronella.
- **Lemongrass Essential Oil:** This essential oil is insecticidal and it's great for getting rid of fleas.
- **Lavender Essential Oil:** Many people find lavender to be a gentle and nurturing essential oil, but it has the opposite effect on fleas.

For Wounds

When you get a wound, of course you want to heal it quickly. However, there are many different essential oils to use that will help in different ways.

- **Tea Tree Essential Oil:** This is an antimicrobial so it's great on wounds, but remember that you shouldn't put it directly.
- **Frankincense Essential Oil:** This is an antiseptic, so it's perfect to eliminate germs. You can apply it to wounds without any known side effects, and it will protect you from tetanus as well as becoming septic.
- **Lavender Essential Oil:** This flowery essential oil will help you take care of a wound as well. It can be applied to burns, cuts, and even sunburns. It'll help to improve the formation of scar tissues and has pain relieving properties.
- **Helichrysum Essential Oil:** You can apply this it pricks, open sores, and wounds. It can help to stop bleeding as well.

For Sleep

It doesn't matter if you have a reoccurring sleeping problem or an occasional issue, these essential oils can help. You can either use these essential oils in a warmer, a diffuser, or even sprinkle them on your pillow.

- **Lavender Essential Oil:** This is the most common essential oil for sleep as it calms you down.
- **Roman Chamomile Essential Oil:** This oil has calming and soothing properties that will help you to become sleepy.
- **Ylang Ylang Essential Oil:** This will help to not only get you to sleep but to help improve your quality of sleep.
- **Marjoram Essential Oil:** This will help you to relax by relaxing your muscle and joints which will help you get a good night's sleep.
- **Cedarwood Essential Oil:** This, as stated before, is great at relaxing you enough to sleep.

For Toothaches

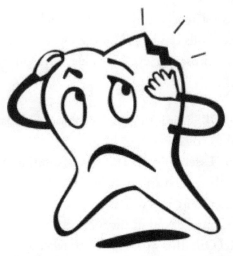

Toothaches happen to the best of us, but you can't always rush to the dentist. These essential oils can help you deal with the pain until you can see a dentist to get to the root of the problem. However, just make sure that you are never putting an essential oil on an exposed nerve. Just place a few drops of the essential oil on a cotton ball and place it near the tooth.

- **Clove Essential Oil:** This is one of the most commonly recommended essential oils to help with a tooth ache, and it will help to numb the area. It's also an antiseptic and anti-inflammatory.
- **Tea Tree Essential Oil:** As an antiseptic and anti-inflammatory it can help with what's causing the pain.
- **Cinnamon Essential Oil:** It can help with the infection and kill of the bacteria that could be causing a cavity. It also helps to reduce the pain by numbing the area.
- **Spearmint or Peppermint Essential Oil:** Both of these have antiseptic properties, and the cooling effect will help with the

pain while it also decreases the inflammation.

- **Frankincense Essential Oil:** It has antiseptic properties while dealing with what could be causing the decay.

Chapter 6: Carrier Oils for Essential Oils

If you've looked into buying essential oils, then you know that they come in small bottles. This is because they're meant to be diluted. The most common size is a 10 ml bottle. A small amount will be more than enough to deliver the health benefits that you need. You can experience adverse effects if you do not properly dilute your essential oils before using them.

Why Dilute Your Essential Oils

You can experience neuro-toxicity, convulsions, headaches, skin coloring, skin discoloration, dermal sensitivity, mucolytic irritation, pre-existing condition aggravation, illness or even death if you do not dilute your essential oils properly. Make sure that you use caution when applying and handling essential oils. Some essential oils are toxic to ingest. These include but are not limited to cassia, horseradish, mustard, Mugwort, rue, saving, tansy, camphor, wormseed, wormwood, thuja, savin, pennyroyal and wintergreen. You'll find a standard dilution guide below.

- **0.25% Dilution:** This is best if you're using it for children that are between six months and six years old. However, you should not use essential oils on a child under the age of two unless you are directed by your doctor.
  - **1 drop to 4 Tablespoons of Carrier Oil**
- **1% Dilution:** This is recommended for pregnant women, elderly adults, sensitive skin types, those with preexisting conditions, or children above the age of six.
  - **1 Drop to 1 Teaspoon of Carrier Oil (5-6 Drops per Ounce)**
- **2% Dilution:** This is the best dilution for most adults. This is good for topical application or aromatherapy.
  - **2 Drops to 1 Teaspoon of Carrier Oils (10-12 Drops per Ounce)**
- **3% Dilution:** This is good for temporary health issues, especially topical application for injury, muscle pains, or even respiratory problems.
  - **3 Drops to 1 Teaspoon of Carrier Oil (1518 Drops per Ounce)**
- **25% Dilution:** Not every essential oil can be used with this

much strength, but there are some that can. There are some essential oils that will not require a dilution. This is good for healthy adults, but you should use this with caution.

- ○ **25 Drops to 1 Teaspoon of Carrier Oil (125-150 Drops per Ounce)**

Carrier Oils

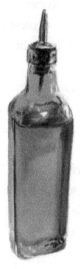

You may be wondering what you need to buy to dilute an essential oil, and this section will tell you everything you need to start blending your essential oils. Carrier oils are natural and come from vegetarian sources. They aren't volatile, which makes them a great medium for dilution so you can use your essential oils. The first thing you need to learn is what a carrier oil isn't.

- Vegetable Shortening
- Margarine
- Butter

These are not intended for topical use, and you shouldn't try to use them as a carrier oil. Don't try petroleum derivatives either, including but not limited to petroleum jelly. Below you'll find what you should use as a carrier oil.

- **Grapeseed Oil:** This oil has a short shelf life, but it's moisturizing. It is great for massages, and it has a thin and light consistency. It's high in linoleic acid as well.

- **Sweet Almond Oil:** This has a nutty and sweet aroma, and it has a medium consistency. It's rich in oleic acid, vitamin E and is moisturizing. This absorbs into your skin quickly, but it will leave a bit of oil on your skin.
- **Olive Oil:** This is popular because it's easy to find. It has a thick consistency and it'll leave your skin feeling oily as well. It's a good source of oleic acid, but it also has a short shelf life. Olive oil has a strong aroma.
- **Jojoba Oil:** This also has a nutty aroma and a medium consistency. It has an absorption that doesn't leave grease on your skin, and it's similar to the natural oils found on your skin. Jojoba oil has a long shelf life.
- **Fractionated Coconut Oil:** This oil is liquid at room temperature unlike most coconut oil, and it has no noticeable smell. This absorbs well, which will leave your skin moisturized and silky. It has a long shelf life while also being high in fatty acids.
- **Coconut Oil:** This is solid at room temperature, so you'll need to heat it up to use it properly. It has a coconut aroma, but the aroma is light. It'll leave your skin moisturized but it's likely to leave a small trace of oil on your skin as well. This type of carrier oil also has a long shelf life.
- **Cocoa Butter:** This is difficult to work with when it's at room temperature, so you'll need to heat it up. You'll need to melt it and blend with other carrier oils for the best results. Cocoa butter has an almost chocolate aroma.
- **Shea Butter:** This is solid at room temperature as well, so you'll need to heat it up to use it. It moisturizes your skin, but it'll leave a waxy feeling as well.

Chapter 7: Skin & Beauty Essential Oil Recipes

It doesn't matter how old you are, you still need to take care of your skin. Sometimes it's to make you look younger, sometimes it's for health reasons, and sometimes it's just so you feel a little better. No matter the reason, this chapter has got you covered.

A Revitalizer Blend

This blend helps to revitalize your skin, giving you a healthy glow that will make you look and feel better. Blend in a carrier oil before applying topically. The carrot seed oil is known to help reduce scars while the frankincense will moisturize your skin, helping to limit wrinkles.

- 10 Drops Frankincense Essential Oil
- 10 Drops Carrot Seed Essential Oil

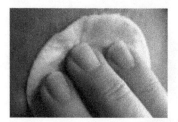

Blemish Reducer

Make sure that you use a carrier oil before applying, but the lavender oil will make your skin silky and soft. The tea tree oil helps to clear blemishes as well. The lemon oil is known to revitalize your skin and help to wake you up.

- 5 Drops Lavender Essential Oil
- 5 Drops Lemon Essential Oil
- 10 Drops Tea Tree Oil

Fine Line Reducer

This blend is known to help you reduce fine lines and wrinkles, helping you to achieve smoother skin.

- 10 Drops Frankincense Essential Oil
- 10 Drops Myrrh Essential Oil
- 5 Drops Goldenrod Essential Oil

Acne Clearing Blend

Everyone has an issue with acne from time to time, but there's no reason to let acne get you down. This blend is perfect for fighting acne, and you should apply it with your carrier oil in the morning.

- 10 Drops Tea Tree Essential Oil
- 15 Drops Geranium Essential Oil

Age Buster

This blend is great for helping you to fight signs of aging, including acne and fine lines.

- 10 Drops Tea Tree Essential Oil
- 15 Drops Neroli Essential Oil

Age Spots & Wrinkle Reducer

Everyone ages, and some people have an issue with age spots more than others. There's no reason to deal with age spots or wrinkles, and when you use this with a lemon then you're sure to find the results you're looking for. Just apply lemon juice and then the essential oil blend along with your carrier oil.

- 15 Drops Rose Essential Oil
- 10 Drops Lemon Essential Oil

Dry Patches & Acne Blend

Rosewood essential oil is a great way to get rid of acne, and lavender will help with dry patches. Just apply topically with a carrier oil as needed.

- 15 Drops Rosewood Essential Oil
- 15 Drops Lavender Essential Oil

Moisture Remedy

It doesn't matter if you have dry skin, oily skin, or both because this essential oil blend is perfect for giving you the balance you need. Just apply it with your carrier oil.

- 10 Drops Patchouli Essential Oil
- 10 Drops Tea Tree Essential Oil

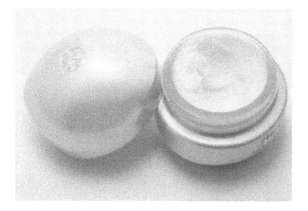

Elasticity Fix & Wrinkle Reduction

Frankincense as well as ylang ylang will restore the elasticity that your skin may be lacking. It will also help to balance your skin and reduce wrinkles as well as fine lines.

- 20 Drops Frankincense Essential Oil
- 20 Drops Ylang Ylang Essential Oil

Clear Skin Remedy

This is a total package essential oil blend. It can do anything from helping to get rid of acne to helping with wrinkles. It can get rid of dry patches or keep your skin from producing excess oil.

- 5 Drops Myrrh Essential Oil
- 5 Drops Lavender Essential Oil
- 5 Drops Ylang Ylang Essential Oil
- 5 Drops Tea Tree Essential Oil

Chapter 8: Stress Reducing Essential Oil Blends

Everyone gets stressed from time to time, but essential oils can help with that too. There are many natural ways to treat stress, but one of the best ways is with a proper essential oil blend. You can use these either topically with a carrier oil or diffuse them.

Using a Diffuser

A diffuser is something that you buy, and it doesn't have to be expensive. You can get a diffuser for under $25. Just make sure that you're using clean tap water, but it can be room temperature. The water level shouldn't exceed where your diffuser marks it. Then all you have to do is turn it on, and let the essential oils do their work. If using the following blends in a diffuser, just add five drops to your water. You can use a warmer instead of a diffuser as well. Just place the five drops on the warmer, and then heat it up by placing a tea light in the warmer before lighting it.

To Revive You

This essential oil blend will help you to feel more awake and ready to tackle on the day while helping to reduce your stress.

- 5 drops Tea Tree Essential Oil
- 15 Drops Vetiver Essential Oil
- 5 Drops Lavender Essential Oil

Clearing Your Mind

When you're stressed out and trying to clear your mind, this blend will help you to do so. This is the perfect blend to use when you're trying to solve a problem and can't seem to think straight.

- 10 Drops Lemon Essential Oil
- 10 Drops Chamomile Essential Oil

Stimulation Blend

This will help to rejuvenate you and stimulate your general senses, which will clear your mind almost instantly.

- 2 Drops Basil Essential Oil
- 8 Drops Grapefruit Essential Oil
- 4 Drops Lemon Essential Oil
- 4 Drops Lavender Essential Oil

Quick Energy Booster

When you feel like you're lacking energy there's no reason to go for that energy drink or a cup of coffee when you can use this essential oil blend.

- 5 Drops Wild Orange Essential Oil
- 5 Drops Peppermint Essential Oil

Quick Focus

When you're having an issue with focusing, then this essential oil will help. Stress is usually the cause, so this helps to heighten your focus while relieving any stress or anxiety you might be feeling. This blend is best used in a diffuser.

- 5 Drops Vetiver Essential Oil
- 5 Drops Frankincense Essential Oil

Relaxing Chamomile

This is a mainly chamomile blend that will help you to relax from stress and depression, but it's best to use this when you don't have to go anywhere. It can make many people feel sleepy.

- 2 Drops Marjoram Essential Oil
- 4 Drops Ylang Ylang Essential Oil
- 6 Drops Roman Chamomile Essential Oil

Easy Sleep

When dealing with stress, it can be difficult to fall asleep. That's where this essential oil helps to come in handy. Its best I applied to your sheets, pillow or in a diffuser close by.

- 2 Drops Ylang Ylang Essential Oil
- 2 Drops Patchouli Essential Oil
- 2 Drops Bergamot Essential Oil
- 2 Drops Lavender Essential Oil

Frustration Reducer

Frustration creeps up on everyone, but this sweet spice helps to keep your demeanor calm even under harsh conditions.

- 5 Drops Orange Essential Oil
- 10 Drops Ylang Ylang Essential Oil
- 10 Drops Cinnamon Essential Oil

Outdoor Stress Reliever

Not everyone is able to go outside whenever they want or enjoy a rose garden, but that doesn't mean you can't enjoy the benefits that would come from one. That's where this essential oil blend comes in handy.

- 5 Drops Cinnamon Essential Oil
- 10 Drops Rose Essential Oil

Lavender Fields

Lavender is known to help with anxiety and stress, but being around fresh lavender can be a challenge.

- 10 Drops Lavender Essential Oil
- 10 Drops Myrrh Essential Oil

Mountain Pick Me Up

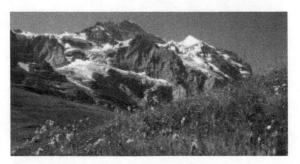

The mountains may not be right around the corner for you, but it'll seem like it with this stress relieving fragrance.

- 15 Drops Goldenseal Essential Oils
- 10 Drops Lemon Essential Oil
- 10 Drops Cedar Essential Oil

Ultimate Rose Blend

If you really like rose sand want a break from the frustration of a hectic day, then you'll find this essential oil blend is great for you.

- 10 Drops Rosewood Essential Oil
- 10 Drops Rose Essential Oil

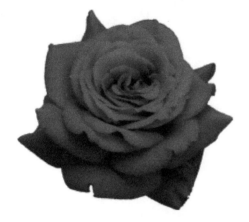

Fennel Pick Me Up

There is no better way to deal with stress than an essential oil blend that will help you to feel more alive and vibrant.

- 10 Drops Rose Essential Oil
- 5 Drops Geranium Essential Oil
- 10 Drops Fennel Essential Oil

Spring in Your Step

If you're missing that spring in your step, then this essential oil blend will do just that. Geranium is known to helping alleviating anxiety, depression and stress.

- 10 Drops Lemon Essential Oil
- 10 Drops Geranium Essential Oil

Chapter 9: Cold & Flu Relieving Essential Oil Blends

When you get a cold, all anyone wants is to get better as quick as they can. Second to that is that they want to relieve the symptoms so that they can feel better while their body takes care of the rest. That's exactly what these blends strive to do. These blends are best for a diffuser.

Cold Relief

This is a basic cold reliever that will help with any coughing that you're experiencing as well.

- 4 Drops Tea Tree Essential Oil
- 4 Drops Cedarwood Essential Oil
- 4 Drops Frankincense Essential Oil

Congestion Clearing

This blend helps to clear your congestion, lift your spirits and help to clear your cold up quickly.

- 5 Drops Eucalyptus Essential Oil
- 4 Drops Tea Tree Essential Oil
- 2 drops Lemon Essential Oil
- 5 Drops Peppermint Essential Oil

Cough Reducing Blend

This blend will help with congestion, but it focuses on reducing cough when healing from a cold.

- 4 Drops Oregano Essential Oil
- 4 Drops Lemon Essential Oil
- 4 Drops Tea Tree Essential Oil
- 4 Drops Peppermint Essential Oil

Revitalizing Cold Reducer

This blend doesn't just help to reduce your common cold symptoms, but it can help with flue symptoms as well. It stimulates your immune system and helps to eliminate your cough.

- 4 Drops Rosemary Essential Oil
- 4 Drops Frankincense Essential Oil
- 4 Drops Eucalyptus Essential Oil

Easy Breathing Blend

One of the worst parts about having the cold or flu is that you feel like you can't breathe. Just don't use this blend before bed as it'll help to wake you up as well.

- 5 Drops Eucalyptus Essential Oil
- 5 Drops Rosemary Essential Oil
- 3 Drops Peppermint Essential Oil

Immune Booster

If you want to kick a cold or flu faster, then you need to try this amazing essential oil blend.

- 4 Drops Clove Bud Essential Oil
- 4 Drops Lemon Essential Oil
- 2 Drops Eucalyptus Essential Oil
- 2 Drops Rosemary Essential Oil
- 2 Drops Cinnamon Bark Essential Oil

Chapter 10: Pain Relief Essential Oil Blends

Everyone experiences pain, but when you have essential oils on hand there is no reason to deal with it. This chapter will address different types of pain and which blends are best for them.

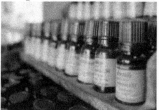

Stomach Pain Blend

This can be used for headaches as well, but this blend is most commonly used across the stomach to help reduce your stomach pain quickly.

- 10 Drops Spearmint Essential Oil
- 10 Drops Peppermint Essential Oil

Joint & Muscle Blend

This will help with any soreness in your muscles or joints.

- 4 Drops Peppermint Essential Oil
- 4 Drops Thyme Essential Oil
- 4 Drops Dark Pepper Essential Oil
- 10 Drops Basil Essential Oil
- 4 Drops Rosemary Essential Oil

Sore Muscle Relief

Everyone deals with sore muscle from time to time, and no matter the cause this blend can help.

- 15 Drops Peppermint Essential Oil
- 15 Drops Clove Essential Oil

Arthritis Pain

Arthritis is persistent, so you might want to grab a roller bottle for this blend so that you can keep it on hand. It may be complex, but this blend will give you the relief that you need.

- 10 Drops Lavender Essential Oil
- 5 Drops Rosemary Essential Oil
- 5 Drops Birch Essential Oil
- 3 Drops Peppermint Essential Oil

Deep Relief

This is good for deep muscle aches that you can't seem to get rid of. It's another complex blend and you might want to grab a roller bottle too.

- 2 Drops Clove Essential Oil
- 3 Drops Vetiver Essential Oil
- 6 Drops Copaiba Essential Oil
- 3 Drops Helichrysum Essential Oil
- 4 Drops Peppermint Essential Oil
- 6 Drops Wintergreen Essential Oil
- 5 Drops Balsam Fir Essential Oil
- 3 Drops Lemon Essential Oil

Nerve Pain

Many people deal with nerve pain, and it can be a difficult pain to treat. It doesn't matter if it's from pinched nerves, shingles, chronic fatigue or a nerve related disorder. This blend can help!

- 4 Drops Roman Chamomile Essential Oil
- 2 Drops Lavender Essential Oil
- 3 Drops Marjoram Essential Oil
- 2 Drops Helichyrsum Essential Oil

Warming Pain Blend

When applied topically, this will help to warm an area and help with minor muscle pain.

- 4 Drops Black Pepper Essential Oil
- 4 Drops Marjoram Essential Oil
- 2 Drops Lavender Essential Oil
- 4 Drops Roman Chamomile Essential Oil

Chapter 11: Miscellaneous Remedies Essential Oil Blends

No matter the reason behind your motion sickness, these topical essential oil blends are perfect to help. Just remember to grab your carrier oil so that you can properly dilute them.

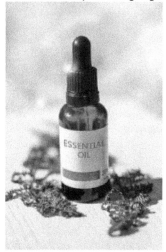

Traveling Sickness

This blend helps to reduce motion sickness from traveling no matter if that's by car, plane, or even a boat.

- 10 Drops Peppermint Essential Oil
- 4 Drops Lavender Essential Oil

Another Immune Booster

This is great for a cold and flu, but its better when you use it as a general boost to your health. The moment you start to feel down, use this essential oil blend.

- 10 Drops Red Orange Essential Oil
- 10 Drops Orange Essential Oil
- 10 Drops Lemon Essential Oil

Pep Me Up

This is another blend that is great when you're feeling nervous about something. It doesn't go as far as to eliminate stress, but it'll make you feel a little less nervous as well as a little more awake.

- 5 Drops Lemongrass Essential Oil
- 10 Drops Peppermint Essential Oil

Cleaning Blend

This blend actually will help you to clean your home. You'll want to put it in a jar with water, and then spray it on your cleaning rag to make sure you don't miss a spot.

- 10 Drops Lemon Essential Oil
- 10 Drops Cinnamon Essential Oil
- 10 Drops Orange Essential Oil

Scar Reducer

This blend will help you to minimize your scars so that you won't see them as much. Don't expect immediate results, but you can use this once a day. You should notice some results within a week.

- 6 Drops Patchouli Essential Oil
- 6 Drops Lavender Essential Oil
- 6 Drops Peppermint Essential Oil

Cheerful Blend

This essential oil blend is another pick me up which will help you to boost your mood no matter the reason you're down.

- 10 Drops Sunflower Oil
- 10 Drops Argon Essential Oil
- 10 Drops Lemon Essential Oil

Stuffiness Blend

This is a blend that will help you to reduce stuffiness in the nose when you rub it under your nose. It will also help with the soreness you experience from blowing your nose too much.

- 10 Drops Sunflower Oil
- 6 Drops Saffron Essential Oil
- 6 Drops Lavender Essential Oil

Focus Blend

This blend will help you to focus a little more when you find your mind wandering, and it can help to improve your mood as well.

- 10 Drops Fennel Essential Oil
- 10 Drops Peppermint Essential Oil
- 10 Drops Lavender Essential Oil

Circulation Improver

This helps to enhance your body's circulation, which can in turn reduce pain.

- 4 Drops Ginger Essential Oil
- 4 Drops Frankincense Essential Oil
- 4 Drops Cypress Essential Oil
- 4 Drops Juniper Berry Essential Oil
- 4 Drops Black Pepper Essential Oil
- 4 Drops Geranium Essential Oil

Vein Blend

This will help with blocked veins or arteries that are causing strain and exhaustion in your muscles.

- 4 Drops Sandalwood Essential Oil
- 4 Drops Neroli Essential Oil
- 4 Drops Sandalwood Essential Oil
- 4 Drops Lemon Essential Oil
- 4 Drops Cypress Essential Oil
- 4 Drops Geranium Essential Oil

Cut Soother

This is good for any scrape or cut you get, helping to clean it out and make it heal a little faster.

- 10 Drops Tea Tree Essential Oil
- 10 Drops Lavender Essential Oil

Menstrual Cramp Reliever

This can be used for any cramps, but this particular blend is best for menstrual cramps.

- 7 Drops Melissa Essential Oil
- 7 Drops Lavender Essential Oil
- 7 Drops Rosemary Essential Oil

Chest Congestion Remedy

No matter why you are having problems with chest congestion, this blend will help you to open up your airways and take care of the clogged area.

- 4 Drops Peppermint Essential Oil
- 15 Drops Eucalyptus Essential Oil
- 4 Drops Ravensara Essential Oil

Antimicrobial Blend

This will help you to clean any cuts or wounds, but it can also be used for skin issues such as acne.

- 4 Drops Cinnamon Essential Oil
- 4 Drops Rosemary Essential Oil
- 4 Drops Thyme Essential Oil
- 4 Drops Lemongrass Essential Oil

Speedy Recovery

This is an antiseptic blend that will help with a speedier recovery as well.

- 10 Drops Lavender Essential Oil
- 2 Drops Lemon Essential Oil
- 8 Drops Rosemary Essential Oil

Sunburn Remedy

This will help to alleviate the pain that you feel from a sunburn, but it also helps your skin to recuperate from the damage as well.

- 4 Drops Lavender Essential Oil
- 4 Drops Chamomile Essential Oil
- 4 Drops Tea Tree Essential Oil
- 4 Drops Peppermint Essential Oil

Varicose Veins

If you want to reduce or get rid of varicose veins, then you'll want to try applying this remedy on daily.

- 5 Drops Cypress Essential Oil
- 5 Drops Lemongrass Essential Oil
- 7 Drops Lemon Essential Oil
- 3 Drops Helichrysum Essential Oil

Chapter 12: Essential Oils for Your Home

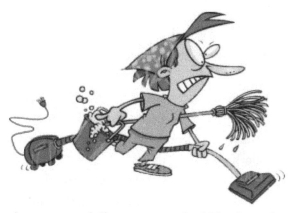

You know many different essential oil blends, and you already know a few cleaning remedies. However, there are many ways that you can use essential oils in your home as well. This chapter will give you even more reasons that you should keep essential oils stocked in your house.

Some Easy Uses

Just follow the directions below.

- **Another Bug Spray:** Use a drop of citronella oil, eucalyptus oil and lemongrass oil. Add it to coconut oil and then rub it over your skin.
- **Sports Equipment:** Add two drops of tea tree oil, lemon essential oil and a quart of water. Add four tablespoons of baking soda, mixing it well. You can use it to clean the odor out of sports clothing and gear.
- **Washing Machine:** If you want your washing machine to smell fresh and make sure your clothe do too, then add twenty drop of wild orange, lavender, or vanilla to your washing machine.
- **Vacuum Cleaner:** If you are having issues with your vacuum cleaner creating a smell whenever you vacuum, you may want to add ten drops of your favorite oil to the bag or dust container that you're using.
- **Soap Scum:** Take a sixteen ounce spray bottle, adding in four drops of tea tree oil, and four drops of eucalyptus to warm water. Spray over the soap scum to kill the mold and scum that is there. You can then wipe it away after leaving it to sit for twenty minutes.
- **Burnt Pans:** There is no reason to throw away those burnt pans when you can salvage them. A few drops of lemon essential oil to boiling water make a great soak for burnt pans, helping to remove the burnt on food after a half hour.
- **Odor Eliminator:** If you want your home to smell better, then diffuse rosemary, orange, and clove essential oils.
- **Pest Control:** Clove oil and orange essential oil can be mixed and sprayed on pests to kill them instantly.

- **Carpet Cleaner:** If you're having an issue with your carpets, borax is an easy fix when you mix in twenty drops of tea tree essential oil. Sprinkle it over your carpets and let it sit for a minimum of fifteen minutes before you vacuum.
- **Mold Eliminator:** If you are worried about mold hanging around in the area, then just add tea tree oil to your diffuser.
- **Tub Scrub:** If you think your tub needs a little extra sparkle and has some bacteria in it that you need to kill quickly and naturally, then take a half cup of vinegar, a half cup of baking soda, and 4 drops lime essential oil with four drops of bergamot essential oil. Let it sit in the tub for fifteen minutes before cleaning.
- **Trash Can Freshener:** Take two drops of tea tree essential oil and two drops of lemon essential oil, placing them on a cotton ball. Place it in your trashcan, and it will detoxify it as well as decrease the odor.
- **Produce Wash:** If you need to clean fruits and vegetables, there's no need to use soap and water because residue can make you sick. Instead, you'll want to add two drops of lemon essential oil to a bowl of water, dipping them in and washing them with the mixture.
- **Fridge Purifier:** If you are having issues with your fridge, especially with odor but also with bacteria, then add grapefruit oil in your rinsing water.
- **Sparkling Dishes:** A lot of people have an issues with spots when they use their dishwasher, but a few drops of lemon oil will help to get rid of those spots with your next rinse.

Chapter 13: Essential Oil Based Beauty Products

With beauty products, you don't have to get synthetic products when you have essential oils at your disposal.

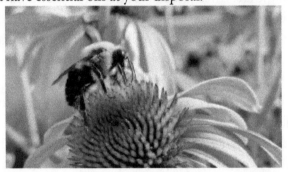

Easy Toner

Toner is great for your skin, and you should apply it gently with a cotton ball once a day after washing and patting your skin dry.

- 4 Ounces Witch Hazel
- ½ Teaspoon Vitamin E Oil
- 3 Drops Cypress Essential Oil
- 3 Drops Lavender Essential Oil
- 3 Drops Geranium Essential Oil

Just mix everything together and put it in a spray bottle. Shake well before each use.

Face Wash

- ½ Cup Castile Soap, Unscented
- 2 Tablespoons Rosehip Seed Oil
- 30 Drops Lavender Essential Oil
- 1 Cup Water

Just mix well and put into a container. It works great with a sixteen ounce foaming soap container.

Face Serum

If you have dry skin, you need some type of moisturizer but sometimes lotion isn't best. Even if you don't have dry skin, a face serum can help you to have a healthy glow to your skin.

- 2 Ounces Carrier Oil
- 20 Drops Essential Oil (according to your skin type)

Cleanse your face, and then apply the serum to your chin, forehead and cheeks. Gently massage in small upward strokes. Store in a glass bottle in a cool, dark place.

- **Essential Oils for Normal Skin:** Lavender, Geranium, Frank incense
- **Essential Oils for Acne Prone Skin:** Cedarwood, Lavender, Tea Tree, Rose, Roman Chamomile, Rosemary, Geranium, Patchouli
- **Essential Oils for Dry Skin:** Lavender, Myrrh, Patchouli, Rose, Ylang Ylang, Clary Sage, Jasmine, Cedarwood, Roman Chamomile, Frankincense
- **Essential Oils for Sensitive Skin:** Lavender, Rose, Geranium, Sandalwood, Jasmine, Frankincense, Helichrysum
- **Essential Oils for Oily Skin:** Geranium, Lavender, Ylang Ylang, Peppermint, Rosemary, Roman Chamomile, Cypress, Sandalwood, Patchouli, Tea Tree
- **Essential Oils for Mature Skin:** Helichrysum, Lavender, Rose, Frankincense, Cypress, Rosemary, Ylang Ylang, Jasmine, Sandalwood, Patchouli, Myrrh

Calming Exfoliating Scrub

This sugar scrub can be used with coarse salt as well, and it will help to rejuvenate your skin as well as exfoliate it.

- 1 ½ Cup Sugar (Brown or White)
- ¼ Cup Coconut Oil
- 8 Drops Lavender Essential Oil
- 3 Drops Purple Food Coloring (optional)

Just mix together and scrub over your skin before washing off gently.

Energizing Exfoliating Scrub

This is a great exfoliating scrub that will help to energize you in the mornings as well.

- ¼ Cup Coconut Oil
- 1 ½ Cups White Sugar
- 10 Drops Lemon Essential Oil
- 2 Drops Yellow Food Coloring (optional)

Just mix everything together and scrub over your skin before washing.

Calming Body Butter

This is a great moisturizer that will also help to calm you down for a good night's sleep.

- 1 Cup Coconut Oil
- 1 Cup Cocoa Butter, Solid
- 10 Drops Lavender Essential Oil
- 5 Drops Jasmine Essential Oil

Directions:

1. Start by melting your coconut oil and coconut butter together over a double boiler.
2. Place in a mixing bowl for thirty to forty-five minutes. It should cool but not harden.
3. Add in your essential oil, and then whip with a hand mixer. It should start to form peaks which will take about ten minutes.
4. Seal in a glass jar, and keep at room temperature.

Essential Oil Shampoo

This essential oil shampoo is great for growing healthy hair and taking care of your scalp. The best part is you know exactly what you're putting on your head.

- ¼ Cup Honey
- 1 Tablespoon Vitamin E Oil
- 2 Tablespoon Coconut Oil
- ¼ Cup Canned Coconut Milk
- ½ Cup Castile Soap, Liquid
- 50 Drops Essential Oils (for your issue)

Just mix everything together and shake before using. Use like normal shampoo.

- **Essential Oils for Universal Healthy Hair:** 20 Drops Lavender & 3 Drops Wild Orange, or 20 Drops Peppermint & 30 Drops Lavender, 15 Drops Lavender & 10 Drops Lemon & 25 Drops Lemongrass
- **Essential Oils for a Flaky Scalp:** 10 Drops Lemon, 10 Drops Tea Tree, 10 Drops Rosemary
- **Essential Oils for Fragile Hair:** 20 Drops Clary Sage, 15 Drops Lavender, 15 Drops Wild Orange
- **Essential Oils for Hair Loss:** 10 Drops Peppermint, 10 Drops Cedarwood, 10 Drops Lavender, 10 Drops Rosemary

Essential Oil Deep Conditioner

Now that you're using the right shampoo for you, you might want to try a DIY essential oil conditioner as well.

- 3 Tablespoons Coconut Oil
- 1 Tablespoon Olive Oil
- 10 Drops Tea Tree Essential Oil

Directions:

1. Mix everything with a hand mixer until it's thick and creamy.
2. Apply to clean, dry hair.
3. Comb through and then let it sit for fifteen to twenty minutes.
4. Rinse, shampoo and style.
5. Repeat once a week for the best results.

Varicose Vein Body Butter

Varicose veins can wreak havoc on your self-esteem, but they can also cause pain. There's no reason not to work on them with this body butter recipe.

- ½ Cup Shea Butter
- ¼ Cup Coconut Oil
- ¼ Cup Jojoba Oil
- 1 Tablespoon Vitamin E
- 10 Drops Lemon Essential Oil
- 5 Drops Fennel Essential Oil
- 10 Drops Cypress Essential Oil
- 5 Drops Helichrysum Essential Oil

Directions:

1. Place your coconut oil, shea butter and jojoba oil together in a double boiler until it is melted and combined. Heat slowly so that your shea butter does not become gritty.
2. Add in your vitamin E, and stir.
3. Remove from heat and mix in your essential oils, blending well.
4. Let it cool down in the fridge, but do not let it become solid.
5. Whip with a hand mixer until it forms stiff peaks.
6. Place in a glass jar and store in a cool, dark place.
7. Use two to three times daily for the best results.

Anti-Wrinkle Cream

Wrinkles are going to happen to anyone, but there's no reason that you need to deal with them. This cream makes it easy to naturally smooth over wrinkles and fine lines.

- 2 Teaspoons Jojoba Oil
- 1 Teaspoon Coconut Oil
- 1 Teaspoon Apricot Kernel Oil
- 1 Teaspoon Rosehip Seed Essential Oil
- 5 Teaspoons Beeswax, Grated
- 5 Drops Carrot Seed Essential Oil
- 2 Teaspoons Rose Water

Directions:

1. Melt your oils and beeswax together in a double boiler.
2. Stir in your essential oil and rose water after removing from heat.
3. Let cool in the fridge, but do not let it become solid.
4. Use a hand mixer, and beat until stiff peaks form.
5. Transfer into a glass jar, storing in a cool, dark place.
6. Use before bed every night after washing your face and patting it dry.

Anti-Aging Night Cream

This is another wrinkle cream that works great overnight. Just remember to wash and dry your face first.

- 1 Tablespoon Cocoa Butter
- ½ Tablespoon Dark Honey, Organic
- 2 Drops Sesame Essential Oil
- 2 Drops Apricot Essential Oil

Directions:

1. Blend together to make a smooth texture and apply every night.
2. Wash off in the morning.

Beard Balm

Men love their beards as much as women love their long hair, but their beard hair is coarser. It can be hard to tame and make look just right, but this beard balm is non greasy and can help to make his beard soft while looking wonderful and manly.

- 2 Tablespoons Shea Butter
- 1 Teaspoon Aloe Vera Gel
- 2 Drops Cedarwood Essential Oil
- 2 Drops Lemongrass Essential Oil

Directions:

1. Melt your shea butter in a double boiler and add in your aloe vera gel.
2. Mix in your essential oils as you take off of heat.
3. Place in a small tin and use once daily with a comb.

Plumping Lip Balm

No one wants to put chemicals on their lips, and that's why there's this natural DIY plumping lip balm that you can use to get that desired plump look. It will also help to improve blood circulation to your lips!

- 15 Drops Cinnamon Essential Oil
- ¾ Tablespoon Honey, Raw
- 1 ½ Beeswax, Grated
- 3 Vitamin E Capsules
- 4 Tablespoons Coconut Oil

Directions:

1. Melt your beeswax in a double boiler, adding your coconut oil.
2. Mix in your vitamin e oil extracted from the capsules and take off heat.
3. Mix in your essential oils, and then mix in your honey.
4. Pour into lip balm containers.

DIY Lip Scrub

Even your lips need a scrub from time to time to bring out their natural color and get rid of dead skin.

- ½ Tablespoon Olive Oil
- ½ Tablespoon Honey, Raw
- ½ Teaspoon Ground Cinnamon
- 2 Rosemary Essential Oil
- 2 Tablespoons Brown Sugar

Directions:

1. Mix together and apply with fingertips.
2. Rub gently until it dries, and then rinse with warm water. You can follow up with the previous lip balm recipe!

Beard Balm #2

Because everyone's hair is different, including their beard, if the other recipe didn't sound up your alley, then try this beard balm.

- ½ Cup Rosemary & Pine Infused Oil
- ¾ Ounce Beeswax, Grated
- ½ Ounce Shea Butter
- 6 Drops Pine Essential Oil
- 6 Drops Rosemary Essential Oil
- 3 Drops Sweet Orange Essential Oil

Directions:

1. Melt your shea butter and beeswax in a double boiler before adding your infused oil. Mix well.
2. Add in your essential oil, mixed well.
3. Store in an airtight container and use once or twice daily before combing through your beard.

Chapter 14: Essential Oil Baths

If you're one of those people that likes to soak in a bath before they get up for work or go to bed, then you'll find that this section is just for you. Essential oils don't have to be made into a cream, salve, used topically or used through a diffuser to have benefits. You can also put different mixtures in your bath in order to get certain results that can help you to get through the week. These bath mixtures aren't hard to make, but to get the right results you'll need to soak for at least twenty minutes so make sure your water is warm!

A Bath for Restful Sleep

It doesn't matter if you're just nervous about something or if you suffer from insomnia. This bath mixture can really help you to relax and get the sleep you both need and deserve.

- 10 Drops Lavender Essential Oil
- 6 Drops Roman Chamomile Essential Oil
- ½ Cup Sea Salt, Coarse
- ¼ Cup Lavender Buds
- 1 Tablespoon Jojoba Oil

A Bath for Stress & Anxiety

Relieving anxiety is important if you want to be productive and get through your week. There is no reason to let stress build up, so try this wonderful nourishing bath for both the mind and body.

- 10 Drops Frankincense Essential Oil
- 5 Drops Lavender Essential Oil
- 5 Drops Bergamot Essential Oil
- 1 Cup Milk, Full Fat

A Bath for Relaxation

This is a stress busting bath, but it works better for a frustrated and stressful day rather than busting up actual depression. Still it can help you to restore your energy after a day that has drained you mentally and physically.

- 10 Drops Rose Essential Oil
- 2 Tablespoons Coconut Oil
- ½ Cup Sea Salt, Coarse
- 10 Drops Frankincense Essential Oil

A Bath for Tension Headaches

This is a great bath for migraines that are caused due to lack of sleep or hormonal problems as well as in general tension headaches.

- 1 Tablespoon Jojoba Oil
- 2 Tablespoons Baking Soda
- 5 Drops Sandalwood Essential Oil
- 10 Drops Peppermint Essential Oil
- 10 Drops Chamomile Essential Oil

A Bath for PMS-ing

If you want to keep your PMS under control, then try this relaxing bath.

- ½ Cup Sea Salt, Coarse
- 1 Tablespoon Jojoba Oil
- 2 Drops Geranium Essential Oil
- 5 Drops Clary Sage Essential Oil
- 3 Drops Chamomile Essential Oil
- 3 Drops Lavender Essential Oil

A Bath for Thought

This bath will help mental fatigue because it stimulates the brain. It can also help with a lack of motivation.

- 5 Drops Basil Essential Oil
- 5 Drops Lemon Essential Oil
- 10 Drops Rosemary Essential Oil
- 2 Tablespoons Olive Oil

A Bath for the Wandering Mind

This bath recipe is great if your mind is wandering of you're having a hard time taking control of your emotions.

- 5 Drops Sandalwood Essential Oil
- 5 Drops Cedarwood Essential Oil
- 10 Drops Vetiver Essential Oil
- 2 Tablespoons Jojoba Oil

A Bath for Preventing a Cold

This is something that will only help if you soak in it as you feel a cold start coming on. However, it can help to erase cold symptoms as well.

- 5 Drops Lemon Essential Oil
- 5 Drops Eucalyptus Essential Oil
- 2 Drops Pine Need Essential Oil
- 2 Drops Tea Tree Essential Oil
- 2 Tablespoons Coconut Oil

A Bath for Bad Allergies

No one likes dealing with allergies, but it can get easier if you have a bath you can relax in that will also take your allergy problems away.

- 1 Tablespoon Sesame Seed Oil
- ¼ Cup Himalayan Salt
- 5 Drops Basil Essential Oil
- 10 Drops Lavender Essential Oil

A Bath for Your Libido

If you're having a hard time rekindling the romance or with your performance, then this bath recipe can help.

- 5 Drops Ylang Ylang Essential Oil
- 5 Drops Sandalwood Essential Oil
- 5 Drops Cinnamon Essential Oil
- 2 Drops Jasmine Essential Oil
- 1 Tablespoon Jojoba Oil

A Bath for Sore Muscles

There will always come a time where you're sore, and no matter what it's for a hot bath will usually work. Of course, this bath will work better than your normal warm water routine.

- 5 Drops Sweet Orange Essential Oil
- 10 Drops Lavender Essential Oil
- 5 Drops Peppermint Essential Oil
- 2 Drops Clove Essential Oil
- 1 Tablespoon Jojoba Oil

A Bath for Headaches

Headaches can be caused for a variety of reasons, but this bath is great at relieving both the cause of the headache as well as the pain that is associated with it.

- 10 Drops Peppermint Essential Oil
- 5 Drops Eucalyptus Essential Oil
- 1 Tablespoon Sesame Seed Oil

Chapter 15: Essential Oil Shower Steamers

Not everyone has the luxury of bathtubs, and some of us are only stuck with a shower. That's where shower steamers come in handy. You'll want to take a fifteen minute shower at least, but these are able to give you the same aromatherapy benefits of the essential oil baths. To use your shower steamers, place them a little bit out of the water's reach. You can sprinkle a few drops of water on them to get them started if necessary.

Your Basic Recipe

The type of essential oils you put in your shower steamers will depend on what you are trying to make, but here is the basic recipe. You can then add the essential oil blend that you want to get the desired result.

- 2 Cups Baking Soda
- 1 Cup Arrowroot Powder (or Cornstarch)
- 1 Cup Citric Acid
- 3-5 Tablespoons Water, Filtered
- Essential Oils

Directions:

1. Start by combining your arrowroot powder, baking soda and citric acid together. You need to make sure that there are no lumps.
2. Add water one tablespoon at a time until you have a consistency where you can make a snowball. It will most likely look dry, but squeeze it and it should pack into a ball easily. If you add too much water, it'll puff up more.
3. Once you get the right consistency, then fill your molds and let them dry overnight.
4. If the molds are still wet they will not fall out easily, but if they are dry they should come out easily.
5. Drop your essential oil blend into each mold. Keep in mind that the blends below are for one bomb.

Congestion Blend

Everyone has that stuffy nose, and you already know that steam can help with congestion in both your chest as well as your nose. Still, with this recipe the steam will help even more than usual.

- 2 Drops Eucalyptus Essential Oil
- 2 Drops Lavender Essential Oil
- 2 Drops Rosemary Essential Oil
- 2 Drops Peppermint Essential Oil

For Your Immune System

As always, boosting your immune system is a great thing. This shower steamer can be used on a regular basis too!

- 1 Drop Cinnamon Essential Oil
- 2 Drops Fir Needle Essential Oil
- 1 Drop Sweet Orange Essential Oil
- 1 Drop Lavender Essential Oil

For Relaxation

Relaxation is important to start your day off or end it after a long, frustrating day. That's where this shower steamer comes in handy.

- 2 Drops Lavender Essential Oil
- 2 Drops Chamomile Essential Oil
- 2 Drops Jasmine Essential Oil

For Focus

This is a great way to prepare for a stressful day, but you can use it after work before you start a project as well.

- 2 Drops Lemon Essential Oil
- 1 Drop Sweet Orange Essential Oil
- 2 Drops Lemon balm Essential Oil

Chapter 16: All about Herbal Tinctures

Before you can learn how to make herbal tinctures, you need to understand exactly what they are. They are the liquid extract that a plant produces, and they're often made in alcohol. However, they can also be extracted in vegetable glycerin, water or even apple cider vinegar. You can use tinctures by placing them right under the tongue so that they are absorbed directly not your bloodstream. This means that the body will be able to react to them quicker. With many herbal tinctures you will notice an almost immediate effect. However, if you are using a nourishing tincture then it can take up to two weeks before you start to notice a difference.

Why Choose a Tincture

There are many great reasons to choose a tincture, but the main one is that they're convenient to use. A month's worth of tincture will usually only be an ounce bottle, which means they're perfect for travel. Tinctures also will help you out in a matter of minutes rather than hours. Many tinctures can be prepared in the comfort of your home as well, and it often comes out to pennies per dose. You also know exactly what you're putting into your body unlike with over the counter medication.

Using a Tincture

You will either get a dosage recommended to you depending on your recipe or you can safely assume it's by the dropper full. This is the quantity that fills the glass pipe on a dropper when the bulb at the top is squeezed and released. These are also often called 'eyedroppers', and they hold about thirty drops. No matter how big the container, they have the same size droppers. Apply the tincture under the tongue so that it gets into your bloodstream as previously stated. Some people will also mix it with honey to obscure the taste of the tincture. You can also mix it with a cup of warm water to make an instant herbal tea.

Chapter 17: Making Your First Tincture

Most tincture recipes, like essential oils, will not tell you an exact way to mix them. This is because the recipe assumes you know how to make the tincture before you begin. That's why this chapter is essential in preparing any of the tincture recipes in this book. Once you know the methods that you can prepare a tincture with, then you'll be able to determine which method is best for you.

The Alcohol Method

This is one of the most popular methods of making a tincture. There are different types of alcohol you can use. Most people stick to 100 proof grain alcohol, which is the most effective, but you can also use vodka, rum or gin as a replacement. After you've chosen your alcohol then you want to chop your plant and put it into a jar. Pour in the alcohol until your plant matter is covered but just slightly. Pour the concoction into your blender, and blend the content. The herb should be pulverized, and your liquid should be milky. Continue blending if you're liquid is too clear. Pour the mixture back into the jar, sealing it tight and then placing it in a warm place. You need to let it sit for four to six weeks.

The Vinegar Method

If you cook a lot then this method works wonderfully because you can use it in cooking as well. When you use apple cider vinegar, then you can get the healing benefits of apple cider vinegar as well. You'll need to prepare your herbs, placing them in a jar with your apple cider vinegar covering them. Blend it, and then replace it back into the container. Remember to leave it for four to six weeks in a warm place.

The Glycerin Method

When you use glycerin, then you'll get a nicer tasting extract most of the time. However, this is the least effective of the three methods found in this chapter. Chop up your plant, placing it in your jar. Next, you'll use a distilled water and glycerin mix, make sure it's 50/50. Pour it over the herbs. Seal the lid, setting the jar aside. If you have harsh winters, this part will be necessary next. Of course, if you live in a climate that is sunny this part may not be needed.

Heat the glycerin extract, and you can do this in several ways. Just make sure it doesn't get near the boiling point. The easiest way to heat it is to place it into a crockpot that's just on the 'warm' setting. You can also put it in an airing cover. Just make sure to keep it there for three to four weeks if you use the cupboard method. If you use the crockpot method, then you'll need to keep it for one to two days. If you just have a sunny climate, you can keep it in a warm spot exposed to sunlight for three to four weeks.

Agitation & Monitoring

You want to shake the tincture jar about once a day for the best results. Over the course of the next few weeks, you should be able to see the liquid go from a milky white to a green to a darker brown. Don't be alarmed by the changing of color, and if you want to help it along you can shake it more than once a day as well. You will also need to top your jars off from time to time. You do not want to top off alcohol or vinegar, and you should use this sparingly.

Storing & Labelling

When your tinctures are done, you're not done with preparing them for use just yet. You'll need a cheesecloth, but a fine mesh sieve or coffee filter would work in a pinch, a funnel, pen and sticky labels. Your tincture will be potent by the time that it is done, but you will need to strain out the plant matter using your cheesecloth, placing it over a sterilized bowl. Use your funnel and place another cheese cloth in it and funnel it into your tincture bottle. You can keep a vinegar or alcohol tincture out, but you will need to refrigerate a glycerin tincture. As far as labeling goes, you should label with the common name, Latin name if you can, part used, fresh/dry, your medium (vinegar, alcohol or glycerin), bottling date, and dose.

Chapter 18: Tincture Myths

Just like with the essential oil myths, there are a few myths that we need to dispel about tinctures as well. This will help you to better understand what you will be using and creating so that you can use it properly. There's no room for misunderstandings when you are using something to address your health concerns.

The Longer Infused the Better

Okay, this one isn't entirely true. You'll find that tinctures do need some time to infuse, but not every tincture is going to get better after four weeks. Most tinctures simply wont get any better, especially when you are using alcohol. You need to let them sit and be patient, but it's not wine. It won't get better with age after a certain point, so there's no reason to waste your time trying to make it stronger by letting it infuse too much longer.

Shaking is an Essential Part

Shaking is essential because you need to make sure it's covered and some of the alcohol will evaporate. For that reason, it's recommended that you shake every day or every other day. However, that doesn't mean that it's going to break down the tincture and help it along to shake it until you nearly break it. You'll just be exhausting yourself for no reason. Agitation is more of an 'in case' type of thing. Don't sweat it if you forget to do it for a few days!

It Has to Be Hot

You don't have to have a hot tincture to make it a good tincture. You can make tinctures in winter, and it'll still be just as potent. It's recommended that it doesn't get cold enough to delay the process, but keeping it indoors will be enough for that. You don't need to worry about placing it in a warm, dark place. All you need to do is just let the tincture be and let the alcohol do its work.

Chapter 19: Popular Tincture Recipes

You can use many different tinctures for the same ailments, but the one you choose should depend on how you react to it, which is trial and error, as well as what is available to you. Arthritis, for example has various tinctures that can be used. Try these popular, easy tincture recipes. Each of these recipes call for alcohol, but you can use whichever method you choose to make your tincture. Never use a tincture if you are pregnant or breastfeeding without talking to your doctor first. Do not use a tincture if you are taking other medications without talking to your doctor first either. Do not give a tincture to anyone under 18 without consulting a doctor first.

Arthritis Tincture

Arthritis is painful and no one wants to deal with it, and relief can come in the most unexpected place. Stinging nettles actually will help to relieve the pain of arthritis or in general joint pain.

- 1 Part Stinging Nettle, Fresh

Take 2 ml three times daily. If you develop a rash or irritation, you need to stop using this tincture immediately.

Immune & Energy Booster

Your immune system is your last line of defense against infection, and it's also your first defense. It's important that you keep your immune system as high as you can, which is exactly what this tincture is supposed to help with.

- 2 Parts Elderberry
- 1 Part Echinacea Leaf
- 2 Parts Echinacea Root
- 1 Part Olive Leaf
- 1 Part Rosehips

Take anywhere from 30-80 drops once daily.

Cardiovascular Tonic

This tincture will help to give you a boost of energy, and it's known to help heart and blood issues. It stimulates your heart to beat.

- 1 Part Ginseng
- 1 Part Hawthorn Berry
- 2 Parts Olive Leaf

Take around five to ten drops every day twice daily. Do not use this with any previous heart medication.

Arthritis Tincture #2

Willow bark has been used in various pain relieving recipes, but it works best for muscular or joint pain. It doesn't help much with nerve pain.

- 1 Part Willow Bark, Dried

Take five to ten drops or about a teaspoon three times daily. You can experience stomach problems if you take more than this. No one under the age of sixteen should take wild willow bark. You should never take white willow bark with ginkgo or vitamin E.

Headache Tincture

Headaches plague many people, and no one likes them. Some people are more prone to them than others, and it can be for a variety of reasons. It can be due to anything from eye strain, to stress to anxiety. This tincture is great when taken alone, but it also makes a great tea to get rid of headaches quickly.

- 3 Parts Lemon Balm
- 2 Parts Feverfew

You should take twenty drops with a glass of warm water as needed. Make sure to not take it more than twice in an hour.

Calming Tincture

Everyone deals with stress, and there are times that you just need to relax. This tincture will help you to alleviate discomfort, stress, and nerve impulses.

- 2 Parts Catnip
- 1 Part Skullcap
- 2 Parts Lemon Balm
- 1 Part Passionflower
- 1 Part Oat Straw
- ¼ Part Hop Flowers

You'll need to take anywhere from one to three dropper full before bed or when you need to relax. Just keep in mind that it can cause you to get tired. If you want to add a stronger sedative effect, then you'll want to add ½ part valerian root. If you still have symptoms after using this treatment for two weeks, then you will want to contact a doctor and stop taking this tincture.

Insomnia Tincture

This is a complex tincture, but if you suffer from insomnia it's well worth it. Sleep is important for your overall health. You can take this tincture in a cup of warm milk as well!

- 2 Parts Chamomile Flowers
- 2 Parts Catnip
- 2 Parts Oat straw
- 2 Parts Yarrow Flowers, Dried
- 1 Part Mint Leaves, Dried
- 1 Part Hops Flowers, Dried
- 1 Part Stevia Leaf, Dried

You should take two to three drops directly under your tongue or a cup of warm water or milk right before bed. Give it about thirty minutes to work.

Arthritis Tincture #3

This can be harder to get ahold of, but it's considered to be a relatively potent pain reliever for arthritis.

- 1 Part Devil's Claw Root, Chopped

Prepare this like you normally would and take about a teaspoon three times daily. You'll want to put this under your tongue for the best results. However, rash is a risk for this tincture as well. Discontinue immediately if you have any symptoms of a rash. Do not use this remedy if you are prone to gallstones. Do not use if you have diabetes or are taking medication as this might affect your blood sugar.

Diarrhea Tincture

No one likes having diarrhea, but this tincture can help you to clear it up quickly if you find yourself suffering from it. agrimony is used because it's an astringent herb which will help to firm up your stool. It also has analgesic, anti-inflammatory as well as anti-viral properties. Thyme is used to relieve diarrhea, and the marshmallow will help to sooth the lining of your gut. Dill, chamomile, peppermint and lemon balm will help to reduce your pain and spasms.

- 1 Part Dill, Dried
- 1 Part Peppermint, Dried
- 1 Part Marshmallow, Dried
- 1 Part Thyme, Dried
- 1 Part Lemon Balm, Dried

You'll want to take this with warm water three to six times daily.

Flu Tincture

This is great during the winter. There's no reason to deal with the cold or flu when you can fight them off. Vitamin C and bio-flavonoids can be found in elderberry as well as rosehips, which will help to fight against the virus. Usnea lichen is great as an immune booster, and it has antibiotic characteristics which will help with respiratory and urinary systems. The mullein encourages your lung's strength.

- 1 Part Rosehip
- 1 Part Elderberry
- 2 Parts Usnea Lichen
- 1 Part Mullein

Take two dropper fulls twice daily, and it's best when mixed with warm water.

Cold & Flu Tincture #2

There's no reason to deal with the cold and flu without trying to get rid of the symptoms. This can help you to feel better while working on fighting off the cause of your cold or flu.

- 1 Part Lemon Balm, Fresh
- 1 Part Horehound, Fresh
- 2 Parts Echinacea Root, Dried
- 1 Part Sage, Fresh

You should start taking this tincture when you start feeling flu or cold symptoms. ¼-1/2 teaspoon of the tincture should be taken every thirty minutes to an hour until you feel improvement in your symptoms.

Athlete's Foot Tincture

This can be an embarrassing and painful ailment. However, it can be easy to treat. One of the main problem is that it is a persistent ailment, but this tincture can help you to get it under control in no time at all.

- 3-4 Teaspoons Cinnamon, Ground
- 3-4 Teaspoons Cloves, Powdered
- 20-30 Garlic Cloves, Fresh & Minced

Once this is made, use a cloth, cotton pad or cotton ball to apply it to your feet, especially on the affected areas. Make sure to also apply it to the area between your toes. You should apply this twice a day, letting it dry thoroughly. After it's dry, try washing your foot with cornstarch. This tincture will need stored in the fridge and used up within thirty days.

Cold Sore Tincture

Cold sores are a pain and no one likes the look of them. Luckily, this tincture can help you to get rid of them while reducing the pain.

- ½ Teaspoon St. John's Wort Tincture (make it or buy it)
- ½ Teaspoon Licorice Root Tincture (make it or buy it)
- 3 Drops Myrrh Essential Oil
- 5 Drops Tea Tree Essential Oil

Apply the tincture directly to the cold sore using a cotton pad or cotton ball. You should do this three times daily.

Healthy Eyes Tincture

One of your most valuable assets is your eyes, and they're put under strain each and every day. Your eyes will strengthen with this tincture, and it can help you to relieve the strain you put them under every day.

- 1 Part Eyebright
- 1 Part Dandelion Root
- 1 Part Nettle Leaf
- 1 Part Fennel Seed

Take twenty drops twice daily with your meals for the best results.

Depression & Anxiety Tincture

If you lack motivation, feel anxious all the time, or feel like nothing is going right you might be suffering from depression.

- 1 Part St. John's Wort
- 1 Part Milky Oats
- 1 Part Skullcap
- 1 Part Ginkgo Biloba

Take a teaspoon three times daily. However, don't expect results right away. It will take time for this tincture to take effect, but you should notice a difference within a month or two.

PMS Relief Tincture

You read that correctly. You can actually make a tincture that can help with PMS symptoms.

- 1 Part Passion Flower
- 1 Part Valerian Root
- 1 Part Pennyroyal
- 1 Part Star Anise
- 1 Part Baneberry Herb

Take thirty to sixty drops in water, and you can take this up to four times daily. Do not take this for more than two weeks continuously.

Sinus Tincture

No matter why you're experiencing poor sinuses, you'll find that this tincture can help to relieve that particular issue or symptom almost immediately.

- 2 Parts Elderberry
- 2 Parts Usnea Lichen
- 2 Parts Oregon Grape Root
- 2 Parts Elecampane Root
- 1 Part Horseradish Root
- 1 Part Yarrow Flower & Leaf

Mix with ten drops of a Cayenne pepper tincture per one ounce. Take two full droppers three times a day with meals, and then take another two before bed for the best results.

Weight Loss Tincture

You'll experience mood stabilization with this tincture as well as better sleep, regular bowel movements, decreased water retention, clearer and balanced skin, and a slimmer waistline.

- 8 Parts Nettle Leaf
- 4 Parts Marshmallow Root
- 4 Parts Senna Leaf
- 8 Parts Eleuthero Root
- 4 Parts Slippery Elm Bark
- 4 Part Dandelion Leaf
- 2 Parts Ginger Root
- 2 Parts Orange Peel
- 2 Parts Sweet Cinnamon Bark
- 1 Part Fennel Seeds

Add a full dropper, adding it to hot water, drinking as tea. It's best to drink for up to eight cups a day.

Chapter 20: All about Infused Oils

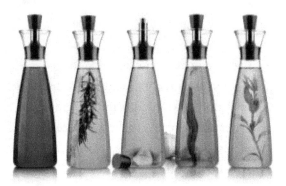

The first thing that you need to know about infused oils is that they are best for ingesting because they do not require you to ingest a high dose. They are not as potent as essential oils, which makes them perfect for cooking with. They can add flavor to your food as well as helping you to get the results that you want. Best yet, they're easy to make at home. The only things that you need to make an herbal oil is the oil that you're using and the herb itself. The rest is just a process.

The Sun Exposure Method

Many people argue that this is a great method to making an infused oil, but it is the most time consuming method. You make it much like you would a tincture. However, instead of using alcohol you'll be using olive oil or coconut oil. Olive oil is recommended because it is more fluid and the night air will not make it turn into a semi-solid much like coconut oil. So, put your herbs in ajar, and then place your oil over them. Fill the jar, and make sure to shake daily. Leave it for one to two months before straining the herbs out and using the oil.

The Skillet Method

Place your herbs in with your oil, and remember that the more herbs you have compared to the oil is best. Though, you will always need to at least cover all of your herbs with some liquid at the top. Thinking of it as boiling eggs. You need to have excess liquid. Heat the herbs and oil together for fifteen to twenty minutes. You can let it simmer, but do not let it come to a boil. Some people will let it simmer softly for an hour for a stronger mixture. Strain out your herbs, letting your oil cool before storing it. This is a little more popular than the sun infusion method because it is quicker, so it'll let you use your oil quicker as well.

Adding Essential Oils

You can actually use the skillet method and add in your essential oils as well. However, the concept of actually ingesting essential oils is up to debate. Keep in mind that not all essential oils can be digested even in low amounts. If you are to add an essential oil to help further the healing properties of your oil, only add two to three drops to every one cup of oil.

Chapter 21: Top Infused Oils to Try

Now that you know how to make your own infused oils, you might be wondering what type of oils to make first. This chapter is dedicated to explaining some of the more common infused oils and what they're used for. The best part about infused oils is not only will they help you with whatever you need, improving your physical, mental and emotional health, but they're a great way to spice up your cooking and baking too!

Rosemary Infused Oil

The best part of rosemary infused oil is that rosemary is a very common herb to use in cooking, so this oil adds wonderful flavor to your meals. It can also help as a memory booster. By consuming rosemary infused oil on a regular basis you'll decrease your chance of developing memory problems at a later age. It can also help to clear up your skin and help you to grow healthy, long hair.

Aloe Vera Infused Oil

Aloe vera is easy to grow, and it grows abundantly as well, making it perfect to use as an infused oil. Just split open one of the leaves and scrape out the 'gooey' stuff inside. This will be the part that you use. You can eat aloe vera, but the taste is up for debate. Still, it's mild enough to go into most foods.

You can use aloe vera infused oil in soap, shampoos, lip balms, or even to cook with. It can be used topically as a moisturizer or even as a massage oil as well. It is full of twenty amino acids, vitamin E, vitamin B1, B2, B6 and vitamin A and E. It has anti-inflammatory effects. It's even an anti-fungal, antibacterial and anti-viral.

Aloe vera contains many antioxidants and has an astringent property as well. It'll promote healthy skin, including skin regeneration after something like a sun burn. You can use this infused oil topically to help with stretch marks, wrinkles, and fine lines. It's a wonderful agent for your hair as well, helping with dry scalp, dandruff and healthy hair growth.

Bay Infused Oil

Bay is another seasoning that is used in the kitchen often, meaning you can cook with it easily and reap the many benefits that come with it. When used regularly bay infused oil can help to improve blood circulation and help to relieve chronic pain. It can also help to prevent hair loss, and it can boost your immune system, helping to keep colds and the flu away. It can also relieve depressive symptoms and improve sleep over time.

Calendula Infused Oil

This isn't everyone's first choice when it comes to cooking, but it has been used since the middle Ages. It was often used to color butter, side dishes and cheeses, and it was even referred to as the "poor man's saffron". Calendula is actually the proper term for marigold. When used topically, infused calendula oil can help with skin issues such as dermatitis, psoriasis, eczema, diaper rashes, acne, bed sores, insect bites and bruises. It can also be used on varicose veins. You can use it internally for chronic inflammation. It's also a great moisturizer so it works wonderfully as a base for lotion.

Dill Infused Oil

Dill is often used in many recipes, so you'll find that it can be used for cooking as well. However, there are many topical uses for dill infused oil as well, especially if you don't have the essential oil on hand. When you use dill infused oil in your cooking it can help with better sleep, and it will help to reduce inflammation. If you rub it on your scalp it can help to protect against head lice as well. It can help relieve stress and anxiety as well.

Ginger Infused Oil

This is another infused oil that is easy to use in the kitchen, and it has a wonderful but pungent aroma. It is known for its anti-inflammatory properties, and it helps to relieve both pain and motion sickness. It can also energize you. It will reduce your risk of blood clots as well as help to decrease cholesterol levels. It can lower your risk of blood pressure issues as well, and it's known to help promote proper digestion and increase your appetite. To infuse ginger oil, you'll need to peel off the outer skin. It'll be easier if you chop the ginger fine so that it'll release its properties into the oil.

Lemon Infused Oil

Lemon is another infused oil that can easily be used in the kitchen, and it adds a nice flavor to your food. It's high in antioxidants and vitamin C as well. Lemon also has calcium, vitamin A and potassium. It reduces inflammation, lowers blood pressure, and helps to address constipation. It will support your immune system as well as soothe indigestion, heart burn and stabilize your mood. You can simply slice the lemon and use all of it to infuse your oil. There are health benefits in the lemon peel as well. If you don't want to use the lemon peel, you can dry it and grate it to make lemon zest to go in your cabinet as well.

Lime Infused Oil

Lime is a great infused oil to use in the kitchen, and it is rich in vitamin C. just like with lemon infused oil, it's a great way to boost your immune system. It calms your mind, relieves stress, fights exhaustion, and helps to address anxiety and depression. You can use it topically to calm frizzy, dull or even oily hair.

You can also use it for acne or other skin conditions. It detoxifies your liver, promotes good oral health by strengthening your gums and preventing tooth loss, and it can help to fight off internal infections. Just like with lemon infused oil, you can use the whole lime to make your infused oil because there are health properties in the peel itself. However, you can also make it without the peel and make lime zest like you would lemon zest. This is a great way to add an additional spice to your cabinet.

Grapefruit Infused Oil

Grapefruit infused oil is packed with antioxidants, and it works as an appetite suppressant. It can be used as a massage oil while also helping to relieve headaches, menstrual cramps, and muscle and joint pain. It can be added to lotions and creams to help with oily skin as well as acne. When you use grapefruit infused oil on a regular basis, it helps to promote a healthy balance of hormones and enzymes. It also helps to promote a healthy digestive function. You can use the whole grapefruit to make grapefruit infused oil because the peel has health benefits as well.

Nutmeg Infused Oil

Nutmeg infused oil is great for arthritis as well as digestive problems. It also helps to address bad breath by eliminating the bad gut bacteria that causes bad breath regularly. It is also is a sleeping aid, and helps to remove toxins from your kidneys and liver. It can help to dissolve kidney stones as well. It helps to treat anxiety and chronic stress as well. When used as a massage oil it can help to relieve muscle pain, treat inflammation and promote good blood circulation.

Parsley Infused Oil

This adds a mild flavor to food, and it promotes digestive health. It can help with arthritis when applied topically but also when ingested over time. It also helps to remove toxins from your blood, which will help to energize you and leave you feeling better overall. Parsley infused oil will also help with chronic inflammation.

Oregano Infused Oil

This is a fragrant infused oil that's great for cooking but it can also be used topically. It helps to relieve sinus infections and colds while boosting the immune system. It can also be used to treat nail fungus when used as a massage oil. It also helps to relieve bug bites, rashes, and helps to sooth a sore throat. It can help to reduce chronic inflammation as well.

Sage Infused Oil

Sage infused oil helps to ward against infections, but it also adds great flavor to dishes. It also works as a laxative, but when used topically it can also be used as a hair conditioner and skin moisturizer. It assists in your metabolic functions, helps to regulate menstrual cycles, helps to regulate hormones, and can reduce toxins in your system.

Sesame Infused Oil

This infused oil is great for Asian inspired dishes, and it's high in omega-6 fats as well. It helps to remove toxins from your mouth, and it can help to prevent diabetes by keeping your blood sugars under control. When used topically it can be used as a natural sunscreen and a moisturizer. It can also help to boost scalp and hair health.

Vanilla Infused Oil

This oil is expensive to make since it requires vanilla bean, but it has many health benefits. Vanilla infused oil can help to relieve nausea and it can help to enhance your libido too. Over time it helps you to get more restful sleep, and it helps to regulate ministration. It works great at speeding up the healing process, relieve anxiety, stress and even fight off depression. It is easier to make infused vanilla oil if you split the vanilla pods before you try to infuse them into your oil.

Thyme Infused Oil

There are many uses for thyme infused oil, and it can help to treat water retention, menopausal and menstrual problems, arthritis, nausea, and even fatigue. It can help with bites, sores, oily skin, athlete's foot and even scars when applied topically. It can also be used as an insect repellent. It is also believed that thyme oil can help to prevent hair loss. It even eases your nerves and deals with anxiety.

Tangerine Infused Oil

Over time, tangerine infused oil can help with weight loss. It also acts as a blood purifier, and it has a calming effect. It can relieve muscle and nerve pain by helping to control spasms as well. Over all, tangerine infused oil is a great way to promote better sleep and improve your mood overall. Just like with the other citrus fruits that you've been using, you can use the whole citrus fruit to make your infused oil. Of course, you can actually save the peel and make a zest in order to bake with it, but you can just bake with this infused oil as well so there's no reason to go through so much trouble. It's all a matter of preference.

Peppermint Infused Oil

Peppermint infused oil is great for cooking, especially if you're making desserts. It helps to reduce anxiety, stress and stave off depression. It's effective in reducing pain, improving your mood, and relieving anxiety. It promotes a healthy digestive system, so it can relieve nausea and stomach pain. Peppermint is also known to help to boost your memory. It also works great at preventing cavities.

Lemongrass Infused Oil

You already know that lemongrass can help to repel insects, but you can also use this infused oil in soaps, shampoos, lotions, deodorants, and cosmetic products. It can help promote a healthy digestive system, prevent infection, prevent hair loss, and reduce chronic inflammation. It can be used topically to promote healthy hair growth by strengthening your hair follicles.

Chapter 22: DIY Herbal Creams & Salves

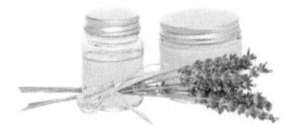

These utilize the same herbs that you use in tinctures as well as essential oils, and they often use essential oils and herbs themselves. Salves and creams can help you with a variety of issues, but they're a little bit more complicated than people think. Still, they're easy to apply and easy to keep track of.

Sleep Deeply Salve

If you're having a hard time falling asleep, then maybe try this salve if you aren't feeling up to a tincture. You can use jojoba oil in place of the grapeseed oil as well.

- 2 Tablespoons Coconut Oil
- 2 Tablespoons Grapeseed Oil
- 15 Drops Lavender Essential Oil
- 15 Drops Cedarwood Essential Oil
- 2 Tablespoons Beeswax

Directions:

1. Start by heating your coconut oil, beeswax and grapeseed oil over a double boiler.
2. Add in your essential oils before stirring.
3. Pour into a glass jar, and store in a cold dark place until you're ready to use it.
4. Rub this salve on your pulse points, and then try to take a couple deep and slow breaths of the scent. It also helps if you rub a little into the soles of your feet.

Sore Muscle Salve

Everyone deals with sore muscles on occasion, and this is a great way to use the essential oils that you have for a good, lasting relief.

- 3 Ounces Beeswax, Grated
- 4 Teaspoons Sweet Almond Oil
- 4 Tablespoons Coconut Oil
- 10 Drops Lavender Essential Oil
- 15 Drops Rosemary Essential Oil
- 10 Drops Lemongrass Essential Oil
- 15 Drops Marjoram Essential Oil

Directions:

1. Melt your beeswax in a double boiler, and then stir in your coconut oil.
2. Add in your sweet almond oil and essential oils, blending well before placing in a glass jar.
3. Apply topically to the area as needed.

Headache Salve

When you have a headache, try this simple headache salve. It's much like the headache essential oil blends you use, but some people find that salves work better. If you don't have peppermint essential oil on hand, you can use spearmint essential oil as well.

- 6 Tablespoons Coconut Oil
- 1 Tablespoon Beeswax, Grated
- 6 Drops Lavender Essential Oil
- 6 Drops Peppermint Essential Oil

Directions:

1. Melt your beeswax in a double boiler, and then add your coconut oil.
2. Make sure to blend well, and then add in your essential oils. Make sure that you blend it well before storing it in a glass jar.
3. Rub it on your temples as needed.

Wrinkle Reduction Cream

No one wants to deal with wrinkles, and you already know that essential oils can help you. However, shea butter and coconut oil makes the perfect carrier with this DIY cream. The frankincense cream is essential for this recipe, but you can replace your lavender essential oil with carrot seed essential oil if you have to.

- ¼ Cup Shea Butter
- ¼ Cup Coconut Oil
- 7 Drops Lavender Essential Oil
- 10 Drops Frankincense Essential Oil

Directions:

1. Melt your shea butter in a double boiler, but make sure not to heat it too quickly or it'll become gritty.
2. Add in your coconut oil, but remove it from heat.
3. Make sure to blend well, adding in your essential oils.
4. Store in a glass jar, and keep it in a cool, dark place.
5. Apply once every morning and once before bed.

Eczema Healing Salve

If you've ever experienced eczema, then you know how painful it can be. This healing salve can help to reduce the pain you feel and help to stop your eczema breakout. Even though this salve is best for eczema, this salve can help with psoriasis as well as common rashes.

- 2 Tablespoons Calendula Infused Oil
- 1 Teaspoon Neem Oil
- 2 Tablespoons Coconut Oil
- 2 Tablespoons Shea Butter
- 1 Tablespoons Beeswax, Grated
- 15 Drops Tea Tree Essential Oil
- 15 Drops German Chamomile Essential Oil
- 15 Drops Bergamot Essential Oil
- 15 Drops Lavender Essential Oil

Directions:

1. Melt your shea butter, coconut oil, calendula oil and beeswax together.
2. Stir in your neem oil, and then add in your essential oils.
3. Make sure to stir well, and then place in a glass jar. Apply as necessary.

Sunburn Salve

Having a sunburn is a bummer, so you'll want to heal it as quickly as you want. That's where this sunburn salve comes in handy. After two or three applications you should notice a large improvement. Even though this salve works best with sunburns, you can use it on any type of burn to help take the sting away and help it to heal faster.

- ¼ Cup Pure Aloe Gel
- ¼ Cup Coconut Oil
- 6 Drops Vitamin E Oil
- 10 Drops Lavender Essential Oil

Directions:

1. Mix your coconut oil and aloe gel together.
2. Add in your lavender essential oil and vitamin E oil, mixing well.
3. Place in a glass jar until you're ready to use it.

Heel Balm

If you're having issues with your feet, such as cracked or dried heals, then this DIY essential oil balm is for you. It's easy to make, but it's even easier to use. It'll help to provide immediate relief as well. You can use this balm on any cracked skin so long as you are not using it on your lips or around your eyes.

- ¾ Cup Coconut Oil
- ½ Cup Shea Butter
- 15 Drops Tea Tree Essential Oil
- 15 Drops Lavender Essential Oil

Directions:

1. Start by melting your shea butter over low heat in a double boiler, making sure to melt it slowly so that it does not become grainy.
2. Add in your coconut oil, blending well before removing from heat.
3. Quickly add in your essential oils and mix thoroughly.
4. Store in a glass jar, and apply up to three times a day.

Scar Salve

Scars can be pesky reminders of accidents, and to everyone wants to deal with a scar for the rest of their life. This DIY scar salve will help to fade your scar to where it's barely noticeable. This scar salve can help to reduce the appearance of stretch marks as well.

- 3 Ounces Coconut Oil
- 2 Ounces Shea Butter
- 1 Ounce Beeswax, Grated
- ¼ Ounce Vitamin E Oil
- 20 Drops Helichrysum Essential Oil
- 40 Drops Frankincense Essential Oil
- 20 Drops Lavender Essential Oil

Directions:

1. Start by melting your coconut oil and shea butter over low heat in a double boiler. Don't melt it too quickly or over stir, or you shea butter can become grainy.
2. Once melted, add in your grated beeswax as well, and then stir in your essential oils.
3. Stir completely before storing in a glass jar in a cool, dark place.
4. Apply twice daily for the best results. It may take up to two weeks before you see a noticeable difference.

Bug Bite Balm

If you're having issues with bug bites, then you may want to soothe away the irritation and speed up the healing process with this easy bug bite balm.

- 2 Tablespoons Shea Butter
- ¼ Teaspoon Calendula Oil
- 1 Ounce Pure Beeswax
- 10 Drops Tea Tree Essential Oil
- 10 Drops Lavender Essential Oil
- 2 Tablespoons Avocado Oil

Directions:

1. Melt your avocado oil, beeswax and shea butter together in a pan and melt. Stir together.
2. Remove from heat and add in your calendula, tea tree essential oil and lavender essential oil.
3. Pour into small jars and apply as needed.

Cold Sore Balm

Cold sores are painful, and this balm can be a little more soothing than applying the essential oils directly.

- 4 Tablespoons Lemon Balm Infused Oil
- 1 Tablespoon + 1 Teaspoon Coconut Oil
- ½ Tablespoon Taman Oil
- ½ Tablespoon Castor Oil
- 2 Tablespoons Beeswax, Grated
- 1 Tablespoon Shea Butter
- 15 Drops Tea Tree Essential Oil
- 2 Drops Clove Bud Essential Oil
- 25 Drops Peppermint Essential Oil
- 1 Vitamin E Capsule

Directions:

1. Combine your coconut oil, shea butter and beeswax in a double boiler, and make sure to melt it at low heat.
2. Prick your vitamin E capsule and empty the contents, adding in all of your infused oil sand essential oils. Stir well before placing in an airtight container.
3. Apply two to three times daily for the best results.

Hand Salve

This hand salve is great for itching, irritated, cracked or peeling hands. It doesn't matter if it's from a harsh winter or a hard day's work. Either way, this hand salve will help. This hand salve will work for irritated, cracked, itching or peeling feet as well.

- 3 Ounces Olive Oil
- 2 Ounces Coconut Oil
- 1 Tablespoon Calendula Petals Dried
- 1 Tablespoon Lavender Buds, Dried
- 2 Ounces Beeswax, Grated
- 2 Ounces Shea Butter

Directions:

1. Start by heating your olive and coconut oil, and then add in your dried lavender and calendula petals.
2. Let sit for thirty to sixty minutes before straining.
3. Add in your beeswax, melting again.
4. Remove from heat before adding in your shea butter, melting quickly and stirring.
5. Let it cool, and then pour into a clean jar.

Bruise Balm

This is a great way to get rid of bruises quickly, and you should notice your bruise fading in as little as a day. Do not use this on open wounds due to the borax. You can use the same mixture on open wounds if you leave the borax out of the mixture as well. Though, without the borax it'll be a little thinner too. The arnica won't just help with healing your bruise but it will help with the soreness and pain as well.

- 2/3 Cup Sweet Almond Oil
- ½ Cup Arnica Flowers, Dried
- ¼ Cup Beeswax, Grated
- ½ Cup Shea Butter
- ¼ Cup Borax, Cosmetic Grade
- 4 Drops Comfrey Essential Oil
- ¼ Cup Distilled Water, Hot

Directions:

1. Add your carrier oil and dried arnica and infuse as you would any infusion oil.
2. Once you've strained it and have the remaining oil, take ½ cup of your infused oil and put it in a double boiler. Add in your beeswax and shea butter.
3. Melt it all together.
4. In another cup, add your water and borax together. Stir until completely dissolved.
5. Pour this mixture into your oil mixture. Once mixed, add in your comfrey oil.
6. Let it cool, and then whip until it forms stiff peaks. Place in a jar and use as necessary.

Poison Ivy Salve

You already know that sage is an astringent, antiseptic and works as an anti-inflammatory. The plantain is also an anti-inflammatory but it has soothing properties too. The jewelweed helps to heal the skin and counteracts the poison ivy. You can double the plantain if you don't have jewelweed on hand. This can be used on insect bites as well as poison ivy.

- 4 Ounces Jewelweed Infused Oil
- 2 Ounces Plantain Infused Oil
- 2 Ounces Sage Infused Oil
- 2 Ounces Beeswax

Directions:

1. Melt your beeswax and oil together in a double boiler.
2. Store in a cool, dark place until you're ready to use it.

Tattoo Balm

Everyone that has ever gotten a tattoo knows how important a tattoo balm can be. Even if this is your first tattoo, you'll want to have this tattoo balm on hand to sooth the irritation and speed up the healing process without damaging your ink.

- 1 Tablespoon Calendula infused Oil
- 1 Tablespoon Plantain Infused Oil
- 1 Tablespoon Oregon Grape Root Infused Oil
- 1 Tablespoon Shea Butter
- 2 Tablespoons Cocoa Butter
- ½ Teaspoon Vitamin E Oil

Directions:

1. Melt your cocoa butter and shea butter in a double boiler before adding in your infused oils.
2. Add in your vitamin E oils.
3. Refrigerate for thirty minutes, and then whip until it forms soft peaks.
4. Store in a glass container until you're ready to use it.

Nursing Balm

If you are new mother and you're nursing your child, then chances are that you have sore nipples. This is a great balm for cracked, sore or even peeling nipples. Just make sure to wash the area before breastfeeding.

- ½ Tablespoon Beeswax, Grated
- 1 Tablespoon Coconut Oil
- 1 Tablespoon Jojoba Oil
- 3 Tablespoons Olive Oil

Directions:

1. Melt your beeswax in a double boiler before adding your oils.
2. Apply twice daily. Once in the morning and once before bed. Remember to wash the area before breastfeeding again.

Allergy Nose Balm

Whenever you need fast relief apply this to the base of your nose and nostrils. You can also apply it on your temples and cheeks. This balm has a calming effect as well, and for many people it'll help them to get better rest even while they're feeling ill from allergies.

- 1 Tablespoon Beeswax, Grated
- 2 Tablespoons Coconut Oil
- 5 Drops Spearmint Essential Oil
- 5 Drops Lavender Essential Oil
- 4 Drops Lemon Essential Oil

Directions:

1. Melt your beeswax in a double boiler before adding your coconut oil.
2. Once it's combined well take it off of heat and quickly mix in your essential oils.
3. Store in an airtight container until you're ready to use it.

Conclusion

You now know everything you need to know in order to treat issues with herbs instead of chemicals and over the counter medication. From infused oils added into your diets to all of the various things you can do with essential oils and tinctures, you have the knowledge at your disposal. Try a few different remedies out, and remember not every remedy will work for every person. You should never add tinctures, essential oils or infused oils into your regular routine without asking your doctor first, especially if you are nursing, pregnant or have preexisting conditions.

Lastly, if you enjoyed this book could you please leave a review on the retailer's website where you purchased the ebook? It will be greatly appreciated. Thanks and good luck!

Kathy Wyatt

www.FunHappyLives.com

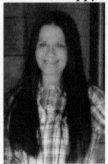

| Page